The Midwife's Tale

About the authors

Nicky Leap was born in 1948 in South London. She has four children, the oldest of whom is 24. She undertook direct-entry midwifery training in 1980 and since 1983 has worked as an independent midwifery practitioner, specialising in home births. Nicky has directed and produced two videos: *Helping You to Make Your Own Decisions – antenatal and postnatal groups in Deptford, South East London* and *Home Birth – Your Choice*. She is co-author of *Your Body Your Baby Your Life* (Pandora Press 1983), and is a speaker at national and international conferences.

Billie Hunter was born in 1953 in South London. She has two sons aged 8 and 3. She worked as a district nurse and health visitor before training as a midwife in 1979. Billie has worked as a midwife in a rural G.P. unit in Brecon, Wales, as an independent midwife in North London, and as a health visitor in the Outer Hebrides, covering remote islands. She currently lectures in Health Studies at Pembrokeshire College, Wales. She has had several poems published in anthologies and a short story in *Everyday Matters* (Sheba Press 1984).

Nicky Leap
Billie Hunter

The Midwife's Tale

An oral history from handywoman to professional midwife

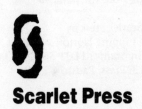

Scarlet Press

Published by Scarlet Press
5 Montague Road, London E8 2HN

British Library Cataloguing-in-Publication-Data
A catalogue record for this book is available from the British Library

ISBN 1 85727 041 X pb
      1 85727 036 3 hb

Designed and produced for Scarlet Press by
Chase Production Services, Chipping Norton
Typeset from author's disks by Stanford DTP Services, Milton Keynes
Printed in Great Britain by T.J. Press, Padstow

Contents

*Photographs of midwifery and birth are between pages
140 and 141*

*This book is dedicated to the memory
of Edie Martinson, Elsie Hunter,
and Lizmiriam Allen, who have
inspired us by their lives*

Acknowledgements

This book has taken eight years to write and has evolved slowly around hectic work schedules and family commitments – including the births of four of our children. First and foremost, we would like to thank all the contributors. They welcomed us into their homes and trusted us with their stories.

We are indebted to Philippa Brewster for giving us the confidence to pursue an idea. In 1991, Scarlet Press saw potential in our unwieldy mass of reminiscences and gave us Gilda O'Neill, whose skill and enthusiasm helped us transform an initial draft into something resembling a book. We learnt so much from her expertise and felt lifted by her wonderful sense of humour and friendship.

Our editor Ann Treneman has been a constant source of encouragement and we would like to thank her for believing in the book. We are also grateful to Vicky Wilson at Scarlet for her guidance and attention to detail.

The following helped us reach people to interview: Barbara Stevenson and Ruth Ashton at the Royal College of Midwives, Helen Adshead, Mary Cuzner, Marcus Grant, Simmy and Gay Viinikka, Dan Wright, Tony Durnford, Margaret and Chris Sparvell, the Borough Community Centre, Charterhouse Pensioners' Group and Field Lane Day Centre. Writers and historians who generously shared their knowledge and gave us encouragement included Brooke Heagerty, Mary Chamberlain, Ruth Richardson, Bob Little, Marion Kozak, Sheila Kitzinger, Jenny Carter and Therese Duriez. Special thanks go to Jan Ayres, Judith Ions and Lesley Moss at the library of the Royal College of Midwives and, also to Trish LeGal from the Independent Photography Project for her advice about finding and selecting photographs.

We have received invaluable help with word-processing, typing and photocopying and have been supported through some nerve-wracking technical hitches during unsociable hours by Don and June Hunter, Audrey Titmuss, Hilary Dunn, Stephen Mak, John Raftery and David and Nogo Confino.

The photographs are reproduced by kind permission of the Hulton Picture Library, the Independent Photography Project, the Greater London Photograph Library, the Cambridge News and the Royal College of Nursing.

All efforts have been made to trace the holders of copyright, but this has not always been possible in the case of some of the older texts. We would appreciate being notified of any corrections or additions.

Finally, the following close friends and members of our families have supported us and put in hours of work servicing us, providing childcare, and bolstering flagging spirits: Katrina Allen, Stuart McHardy, Annie Scotland, Hester Lean, Reuben Turkie, Moyra Weston, Mike Layward, Sarah Maltin, Lizmiriam Allen, Rosalind Stopps and Tina Heptinstall.
N.L. and B.H.

Introduction

In the 1990s in Britain, midwifery is a profession open to women of all social classes and backgrounds, but this has not always been the case. In the early part of this century the profession was restricted to women who could afford the training, in terms of both money and opportunity. A successful campaign to professionalise midwifery was in operation, spearheaded by socially influential, aristocratic and middle-class women whose aim was to build a new profession for women and eradicate the practice of the working-class lay midwife – the 'handywoman'.

The campaigners asserted that professional midwifery would reduce the appalling rate of infant and maternal deaths. As the testimonies in this book reveal, another pregnancy was often something to be dreaded at a time when poverty imposed a lifetime of struggle and hardship for so many people.

The authors of this book are also both midwives. We have used original interviews and secondary research to weave together vivid, often moving stories of midwives, handywomen and the women they attended in the days before the National Health Service.

Although the experience of childbirth could be harrowing for both mother and midwife, the strength and tenacity of the women involved shines out in their accounts of their lives and experiences.

The book begins by looking at the evolution of the profession of midwifery and the demise of the handywoman. This is followed by an exploration of the lives of handywomen as remembered by their children, by the mothers they attended and by the professional midwives who succeeded them.

It is rare to find a handywoman alive today in Britain. They tended to be elderly when they were practising at the beginning of the century, and their traditional skills – midwifery, laying out the dead and tending the sick – faded into extinction as such tasks became institutionalised within a state-run health service. It was, therefore, an unexpected privilege to find Mrs G., a 95-year-old handywoman who was prepared to talk to us and describe her working life.

Next, the book explores the training and working lives of the new professional midwives who took the place of the handywomen. Most of them worked 'on the district' in an age when the majority of babies were born at home. They saw midwifery as a vocation and describe the dedication that was necessary when they were on call 24 hours a day with little, if any, off-duty time. In the words of Dr Janet Campbell, Senior Medical Officer at the Ministry of Health throughout the 1920s:

> The work of a busy midwife is very hard, holidays and off-duty times are difficult to secure, the responsibility is exceptionally grave, the remuneration comparatively small. Midwifery, more than any other branch of nursing, unquestionably taxes to the utmost professional skill and judgement, physical capacity and endurance, patience and sympathy. [Report on the Physical Welfare of Mothers and Children, England and Wales 1923]

Subsequent chapters of the book explore the context within which midwives worked during this era. In particular, the lack of sex-related information and women's low expectations of sexuality are explored. Women describe a time when contraception was unavailable for the vast majority, abortion was a common method of fertility control, and single parenthood often meant social isolation.

Women also talk about how their work, whether paid or in the home, affected their physical and emotional health. Working-class women recall lives of drudgery and exhaustion, where each pregnancy brought increasing poverty and the possibility of bereavement. The situation was not to improve until the Second World War, when concern for the state of the nation's health brought about a new system of welfare benefits. This led to a dramatic reduction in both infant and maternal mortality figures. During the war, midwives had to adapt their practice to cope with the disruption of evacuation and air-raids. They describe how everyone 'rallied round', and how they saw themselves as the mainstay of the community while the men were at the front.

The book concludes with mothers' and midwives' accounts of their experiences of birth. Midwives describe the details of their practice at a time when they were able to offer complete continuity of care and utilise all of their skills.

In the postscript, three quotations pay tribute to the tenacity and courage of many women who gave birth in the first half of this century, and to the midwives who attended them. The inclusion of this tribute reflects a journey we have made since we began the interviews in the mid-1980s.

As can be seen in the chapter entitled Methodology, we had somewhat romantic expectations about our midwifery heritage when we set out to research this book. We expected to uncover a treasure chest of forgotten skills: experiences that would enhance midwifery practice and inspire the midwives of today.

Disappointed by the rigid and authoritarian attitudes that often accompanied the professionalisation of midwifery, we decided that the key to reclaiming the art of midwifery must lie with the much-maligned and persecuted handywoman. Again, we were disappointed. Women described equally disturbing experiences of being at the mercy of authoritarian behaviour from handywomen. There were also accounts that highlighted meddlesome, even dangerous practices, that sometimes took place in the absence of education, where there was limited access to information about the basic anatomy and physiology of childbirth.

The word 'midwife' is derived from the Old English *mid wyf*, meaning 'with woman'. Increasingly, it became clear that the roots of building a new woman-centred midwifery do not necesssarily lie in our recent past. However, over the years that it has taken for this book to evolve, our own attitudes towards the midwives and handywomen who worked in the first half of this century have changed and softened. As we gained more insight into the context of their lives and times, we began to appreciate the extraordinary achievements of these women in the face of severe restrictions imposed by the politics of gender, class and poverty.

The concept of woman-led midwifery care has been developed in recent years within a culture that acknowledges certain egalitarian principles that were unheard of in the early 1900s. However, today's midwives share with their predecessors a passion for the work we do. Many of us will identify with the spirit of early midwifery campaigners. The ideology and language may have changed, but our motivation is common – the commitment to improving the services offered to childbearing women.

Nicky Leap
Billie Hunter
London, December 1992

Who's who: midwives, mothers and others

Midwives interviewed

Edie B.
Born 1894; died 1990.
The eldest of eight children in a working-class family, Edie B. trained as a midwife in Newcastle in 1921. She moved south to Lambeth, where she worked in a maternity home for 50 years. We interviewed her in 1985.

Elsie B.
Born 1906.
Elsie B. trained as a midwife (direct entry) in 1929 in Plymouth. She was a district midwife in rural Devon for the County Council all her life.
We interviewed her in 1985.

Elizabeth C.
Born 1905 in Eire.
Elizabeth C. came from a working-class background and trained in Bradford in the 1930s. She worked as a district midwife in Battersea for many years and was known as 'Auntie Betty' to her clients.
We interviewed her in 1986.

Bronwen H.
Born 1897; died 1988.
Bronwen H. grew up in Swansea, South Wales, and apart from her midwifery training in London in 1921, she spent all her working life there. The third of six children, she trained as a nurse in 1919. She worked as a district nurse/midwife in the docklands area of

Swansea. She gave up this work after marrying the local G.P., since it was not considered 'proper' for the doctor's wife to continue in such a job.
We interviewed her in 1985 and 1987.

Nellie H.

Born 1889 in a Kent village; died in the late 1980s.
Nellie H. trained as a midwife in 1926. She then went to an Essex seaside town to run a private nursing home with her sister Rose. They lived together until Rose died in 1973. Apart from running evacuation programmes for pregnant women during the war, her midwifery career was spent in private nursing homes.
We interviewed her in 1985.

Elsie K.

Born 1904 in a Lancashire town.
Elsie K., daughter of a congregational minister and a teacher, trained as a midwife in 1935 in Derby. She worked mostly in hospital but also undertook some private cases with wealthy families, 'living in' before and after the birth. She later became a midwife tutor.
We interviewed her in 1986.

Katherine L. and Margaret A.

Sisters who were born into a middle-class family in Bromley, Kent, Katherine L. and Margaret A. defied family pressure to become 'professional women' by taking up nursing and, later, midwifery. They eventually worked together as district nurse/midwives in a small Essex town.
We interviewed them in 1985.

Josephine M.

Born 1906 in Sligo, Eire.
Josephine M. came to England in 1906 and has been here ever since. In 1928 she trained as a nurse, followed by midwifery training in London. Initially, she worked in a small maternity home in West London, but then worked on the district in various London boroughs.
We interviewed her in 1986 when she was still doing 'monthly nursing' – living-in postnatal care – for wealthy London families.

Esther S.

Born 1916 in Portsmouth.

Deprived of educational opportunities in her schooling, Esther S. was able to train first as a nurse and then as a midwife during the war. Apart from an initial spell in a small maternity hospital, Esther S. worked as a district midwife in the working-class area where she grew up. She continued to work as a district midwife after having children.

We interviewed her in 1985 and 1992.

Mollie T.

Born 1923 in Bombay, India.

A retired midwifery tutor from a middle-class background, Molly T. worked in London teaching hospitals, local authority and provincial hospitals.

We interviewed her in 1982.

Florence W.

Born 1909; died 1992.

Daughter of a handywoman, Florence W. grew up in impoverished conditions in Great Yarmouth. She was 'rescued' by the Salvation Army, who trained her in nursing and midwifery in the early 1930s. She worked in various Salvation Army hospitals and homes for unmarried mothers and their babies and was promoted to the rank of Brigadier.

We interviewed her in 1987.

Mary W.

Born 1908 in a Yorkshire mining village.

Mary W., a miner's daughter, trained as a midwife in 1931 and returned to the Yorkshire village where she grew up in order to practice as an independent midwife. After 1936, she was employed by the Local Authority and continued to practice in the same village all her working life (37 years), including after she married a winder at the pit and after she had a child. She retired in 1968, having attended the births of 2,002 babies.

We interviewed her in 1986.

Mothers interviewed

Ruby C.

Born 1900 in Belfast, Northern Ireland.

Ruby's father was an engineer; her mother was a court dressmaker. She married a policeman in 1917, and between 1918 and 1924 she had four babies, all born at home in Ireland.

We interviewed her in 1984.

Ivy D.

Born 1904 in south-east London.

Ivy has lived all her life in south-east London. She had four children between 1927 and 1946. Her husband was in the building trade and she owned and ran several shops including a florist's. Later, she and her husband bought and ran a country club in the suburbs of London.

We interviewed her in 1992.

Alice F.

Born 1903 in Dulwich, south London.

Alice's father was a surveyor and her mother's family had a hotel in the home counties. They were a well-off, middle-class family. She had one son by Caesarean section in 1937.

We interviewed her in 1986.

Hannah H.

Born 1901 in London.

Born into a Jewish East End family, Hannah was one of three children. Her father was a tailor's cutter and her mother was a home dressmaker. They were reasonably well-off, lived in West Hampstead and had a maid. She left school at 14, went into office work and later worked for an estate agent. Her husband was a tailor and she had two babies in 1928 and 1937.

We interviewed her in 1986.

Edie M.

Born 1902 in London; died in the early 1990s.

Edie came from a working-class home. Her father was a market-stall holder and her mother was in service. She married in 1920 and had five babies between 1920 and 1935. Two of them died in early infancy. Edie had various jobs throughout her life, including washing-up, waitressing, cooking and factory work. We interviewed her in 1986.

Lou N.

Born 1912 in the Angel, London.
Lou's parents separated so she was brought up by a 'Mrs Amos'. She married in 1931. Her first child, a boy, was born in 1931 and died when he was nine months old. Between 1934 and 1942 she had three daughters. Her various jobs included being a coil-winder, french polisher, brush-maker and office cleaner. We interviewed her in 1986.

Sissy S.

Born 1906 in Deptford, south-east London.
Sissy S. had four babies in the 1930s, with midwife Elsie Walkerdine in attendance.
We interviewed her in 1986.

Jane W.

Born 1902 in Bermondsey, south London.
Jane was one of 14 children and her father was a tanner. Her mother, a laundress, died when she was four, and Jane was brought up by an aunt. In 1923, she married a clerical worker and had two babies, one in 1924 and the other during the war. She worked as a machinist with the Army and Navy Territorial Outfitters.
We interviewed her in 1986.

Vera W.

Born 1903 in Hartlepool, County Durham.
Vera came from a middle-class family. Both her father and her husband were in the building trade. She was one of three children and the family emigrated to Australia in 1909, returning in 1920. She was married in 1934 and had one child by Caesarean section in 1936.
We interviewed her in 1986.

Others

Granny Anderson

A handywoman in Tyneside, remembered by Molly B. and Lily N.

Mrs G.

Born 1894; died 1991.
Born in east London, the ninth of 18 children and daughter of a trained midwife, Mrs G. was a handywoman in the London Borough of Bexley for over 50 years. Mrs G. had eight children – seven boys and a girl who died from meningitis at the age of two. Neighbours called her to attend births, lay out the dead and take care of injuries.
We interviewed her in 1990.

Lily N. and Molly B.

Born 1919 and 1921.
Sisters who grew up in dockland Tyneside, they remember Granny Anderson, the local handywoman, and life in the working-class community there.
We interviewed them in 1988.

Mabel P.

Born 1892; died in the mid-1980s.
Mabel's father was a civil servant, and she grew up in Cork, southern Ireland. The second of six children, she moved to Bristol at the age of 18. She applied to do medicine before women were accepted and so trained as a midwife instead. After working as a district midwife in a Somerset village for a couple of years, she reapplied to Bristol to do medicine and was accepted. On qualification she specialised in obstetrics and gynaecology.
We interviewed her in 1982.

Ma Sturgess

A handywoman in Portsmouth, remembered by midwife Esther S.

Mary T.

Born 1912 in Deptford, south-east London.
Mary worked on the trams, as a fitter during the war and in a biscuit factory. In 1940, she went to live with a sister who lived next door to midwife Elsie Walkerdine. On Christmas Day 1940,

she was invited in to play cards. She stayed the night as no one was in at her house and she never went back to live with her sister. 'Elsie's aunt and uncle cooked for us and when they died in 1952 and 1955, Elsie cooked for me – I wasn't no cook.' Elsie retired in 1957. Mary often went to births with Elsie. She lived for Elsie: 'I never went anywhere without Elsie. I looked on her as like my mum. On the tenancy I was down as her niece.' We interviewed her in 1987.

Alice W.

Born 1884; died 1958.
A handywoman who lived in great Yarmouth, Alice W. had 13 children, 3 of whom died. Her story is told by her son, Ken, in Chapter 2.

Ken W.

Florence W's brother; died 1991.
Interviewed in 1987 regarding his mother Alice. Ken was a nurse. He lived near Reading and had four children.

Elsie Walkerdine

Born 1892; died 1979.
Elsie Walkerdine attended the births of over 4,000 babies in Deptford, south-east London. Until 1937, she worked independently and then for the London County Council. Elsie's mother died soon after she was born. She was brought up by an uncle and aunt who doted on her and saved up for her midwifery training. Before this, Elsie was a needlewoman – 'sewing rich people's cloaks'. She retired in 1957 and is remembered here through the reminiscences of Mary T. and Sissy S.

1 From handywoman to midwife: the development of a profession

Before the First World War and, in some areas, until the mid-1930s, the majority of working-class women in Britain were attended in childbirth not by a professional but by a local woman. She was likely to be an older woman, a respected member of the community. Her role would often include looking after the sick and dying and laying out the dead. Sometimes she also provided a sort of 'home-help' service, taking in washing and helping with housework and childcare.

Today we tend to refer to the traditional childbirth attendant as 'the handywoman', but women whom we interviewed either referred to her as 'the woman you called for' or gave her the title by which she would have been known for centuries – 'the midwife'. Indeed, before legislation placed midwifery firmly in the hands of professionals, the main focus of the handywoman's work was that of midwifery. Childbirth was not seen as a medical process, and in working-class areas, doctors were rarely called for, except in severe emergencies, since people could not afford to pay their fees. As Molly B., who grew up in South Shields, Tyneside, explains:

> We very seldom called for a doctor because you had to pay for it. Everyone was so hard up, you just couldn't afford a doctor. I mean, the only time you were ever taken to hospital was when you were blinkin' on your death bed! The last knockings, you know! [laughter]

In Flora Thompson, in her book *Lark Rise to Candleford*, describes a rural midwife at the end of the last century:

1

She was, of course, not a certified midwife; but she was a decent, intelligent old body, clean in her person and methods and very kind.

Complications at birth were rare; but in the two or three cases where they did occur during her practice, old Mrs Quinton had sufficient skill to recognise the symptoms and send post haste for the doctor. No mother lost her life in childbirth during the decade.

In these more enlightened days the mere mention of the old, untrained village midwife raises the vision of some dirty, drink-sodden old hag without skill or conscience. But not all of them were Sairey Gamps [Charles Dickens's notorious birth attendant in *Martin Chuzzlewit*]. The great majority were clean, knowledgeable old women who took a pride in their office. Nor had many of them been entirely without instruction. The country doctor of that day valued a good midwife in an outlying village and did not begrudge time and trouble in training her. Such a one would save him many a six- or eight-mile drive over bad roads at night, and if a summons did come, he would know that his presence was necessary.

The trained district nurses, when they came a few years later, were a great blessing in country districts, but the old midwife also had her good points for which she now receives no credit. She was no superior person coming into the house to strain its resources to the utmost, and shame the patient by forced confessions that she did not possess this or that, but a neighbour, poor like herself, who would make do with what there was, or, if not, knew where to send to borrow it.[1]

Flora Thompson hints at class barriers and gives an impression of the impact of the predominantly middle-class, certified midwives, when she uses words such as 'superior', 'strain', 'shame' and 'forced confessions'.

In the first decades of this century, an elite group of philanthropic women from middle-class, upper middle-class and aristocratic backgrounds spearheaded a campaign to regulate the training and practice of midwives. They had formed the Midwives Institute in 1881, and under its auspices, they used the political muscle of their connections with social reformers, politicians and the medical profession to manoeuvre the First Midwives Act in 1902. The act was negotiated within a firm understanding that all cases that were not strictly 'normal' should be referred to doctors, thereby ensuring a steady income for the medical profession and minimalising any professional threat to it.

The Midwives Institute aimed to ensure that all women, rich and poor alike, had access to both a qualified midwife and a doctor. Articles in *Nursing Notes*, the journal of the Midwives Institute, describe how their authors also sought to reform working-class habits and values. Central to their campaign was the wish to drive out the handywomen, whom they saw as a source of great evil and danger to childbearing women because they were untrained and had no academic knowledge about the prevention of infection.

The aim of the Midwives Institute was to replace the handywomen with trained professionals drawn from their own ranks. There was also the attraction of creating new opportunities for women at a time when few professions were open to them. Midwifery offered the possibility of responsible work with practitioner status, in a field where there was limited direct competition with men. Undoubtedly, the pioneers of the midwifery profession also saw themselves as the saviours of the poor. Alice Gregory, daughter of the Dean of St Paul's, demonstrates in her writing the almost missionary zeal and imperialist fervour with which they approached their campaign:

> Whether the work is taken up by women who love their country and desire the progress of the race, or merely by ignorant self seekers who hope by banding together to exploit working women at their leisure – all this is now hanging in the balance and depends in a measure on the actions of every one of us. While this is so, let no one complain that life has lost its zest or the present time its romance.[2]
>
> Our bodies are active enough, they run, they lift, and get very tired, and then we feel satisfied that we have done our duty, and spent a useful day, but we won't look deeper to see the world as it really is. A great battlefield – on one side principalities and powers, the rulers of darkness, spiritual wickedness in high places. The devil, sending out his emissaries, superstition, dirt, germs that bring disease, taking advantage of the superficiality and carelessness of the nurse, the ignorance and laziness of the mother – all the powers on that side fighting for their existence. And on the other, the Kingdom of God, coming, irresistibly coming,

because God is stronger than the devil, but by virtue of His self-imposed limitations – hindered, set back, delayed in its coming by every one of us, every time we do our work in a perfunctory manner without real purpose and whole heartedness of endeavour.[3]

The First Midwives Act of 1902 instigated the Central Midwives Board (CMB). The Board formulated restrictive practice requirements, a powerful supervisory apparatus and a plenary system, all of which were successfully designed to make it impossible for working-class midwives to continue to practice in the long term.

All midwives who had a recognised qualification in midwifery, either from the London Obstetrical Society or from certain lying-in hospitals, could enrol on the register of qualified midwives. Women who had been in practice for at least one year and who could show proof of good character by producing a reference from their clergyman, could also apply for admission to the Roll. They were known as the *bona fides* and were accepted by the authorities as a stop-gap measure in order to cover a temporary shortage of midwives.

All other women who wanted to practise as midwives had to pass an examination in competence before a certificate would be issued to them. The cost of training was far beyond the means of most working-class women, and the language used in the examination, such as medical Latin, made it impossible for all but the highly educated to pass. A sobering account of the shame and humiliation experienced by a working-class midwife, Mrs Layton, who failed the examination, can be found in *Life as We Have Known it – by Co-operative Working Women*:

> Several doctors advised me to go in for midwifery, but I could not go into hospital for training. The fees were a bar to me. I found that the cheapest training I could get would cost anything from £30 to £50, and then I would have to be away from home for three months. This was quite impossible for my husband's health needed all the care I could bestow on it to keep him anything like fit for work part of his time. I had no money, only as I earned it week by week, and it was impossible to save.
>
> The doctors trained me and sent me up for examination in midwifery. But alas! I failed, as about 130 did at the same examination. The written examination took place at 9pm in a closely packed room. We had two hours to answer the

questions, and a fortnight later an oral examination. It was just five minutes past 10pm when I went into the examiners' room; at ten minutes past I came out with a slip of paper to give the secretary with the word 'failed' written on it. I was told I could pay another fee and go through another exam, but I refused to do so. I was always a little nervous when writing or answering questions, and when I had to do both in a room full of doctors, I felt I should not make a better job of another exam. When the Midwives Act became law, I was recommended for a certificate as a *bona fide* midwife. I have never let anyone see my certificate.[4]

Legislation also laid down rules concerning the equipment and clothing considered essential for safe practice. In 1905, the journal of the Midwives Institute, *Nursing Notes*, published an article that estimated that the cost of the required equipment and lined midwifery bag would be approximately one guinea – a prohibitive amount for most handywomen, especially as many of them were paid in kind.

The rules laid down in the Midwives Act were enforced by a strict method of supervision. Local dignatories, many of whom were not trained in midwifery, medicine or nursing, were appointed to investigate the practice of midwives in their area. In reality, this often meant an invasion of the working-class midwife's privacy. Value judgements made about her life-style at best may have made her feel humiliated; at worst, they threatened her livelihood. Midwives' homes were inspected and expected to be spotlessly clean, but the midwife was warned not to carry out cleaning duties herself to avoid making chapped or traumatised hands a potential source of infection:

> She should be sure that she lives in a healthy house, that her rooms are clean and well ventilated and the drains in order… The midwife…should avoid very rough work such as scrubbing, grate-cleaning or polishing. If she has to do much work of this sort it is wise to wear housemaids' gloves.[5]

A sympathetic inspector writing in *Nursing Notes* about the difficulties of inspecting midwives, had this to say:

> It is obviously impossible for some of these *bona fide* midwives to comply with some of the rules. To begin with, some of them cannot read or write. We cannot teach them

to do this, and it follows, of course, that they cannot take notes or read a thermometer, or indeed be trusted to give accurate details of any of their cases. Some are too poor to get the necessary cotton dresses, or the simplest things for their bags, some have always been dirty, and probably always will remain so, while some appear to drink, though they never seem to be so fuddled that they cannot do their work. It puzzles me to think how some of these ever got on the register at all, but I have found that their cases do as well as the others, and they are often great favourites with their patients... How are we to insist on these ignorant women carrying the things in their bags that are required by the Act? The douching apparatus that they could not use, and which might be a real source of danger if they attempted to do so, the catheter, and many other things that in unskilled hands are so risky?

Some of these country midwives are very kind, and have been doing their work honestly and unselfishly for years.

It is interesting, in any case, to note that a great many of the old midwives, who are now on the register, are not in any way scared by the new Act into running away from a friend in her time of need, be it a real emergency or not, and I have a distinct recollection of a regular virago standing before me at her cottage door, arms akimbo, and a face full of wrath, as she exclaimed, 'Well, the proper midwife wouldn't come so far, and I wasn't going to see a poor thing lie and die![6]

It was not just standards of hygiene that were of concern. Reports from the Plenary Board show that midwives were often struck off the register for not complying with middle-class standards of morality. For example, midwives who were reported for having given birth to children outside of marriage had their certificates immediately revoked.[7]

Campaigners such as Alice Gregory continued to pour scorn on the *bona fides* in subsequent years:

A large number of the old Gamps consented to enrol themselves as certified midwives and continued to deal out death and destruction as they had done in the past, only now under the aegis of the Government.[8]

Charles Dickens's colourful image of Sairey Gamp[9] – sloppy, dirty, drunkard and hired attendant of the poor – was used time and again as a title to discredit the handywomen. They were not in a position to defend themselves, since they were often illiterate and certainly without a voice in the upper echelons of society.

Under the Midwives Act of 1902, after 1910 no person could 'habitually and for gain' attend a woman in childbirth except under the direction of a doctor, unless she was a certified midwife. (For an overview of the various Midwives Acts see the appendix Milestones in Midwifery, pages 198–203.) Many doctors, particularly those working in rural areas where there were no certified midwives, continued to give the handywomen official cover. There was loose interpretation of the words 'under the direction of a doctor', which meant that in reality the doctor was rarely called to a birth except in an emergency. A government report of the time demonstrates that this situation did not go unnoticed:

> It is unfortunately true that certain medical practitioners are willing to work with handywomen as midwifery assistants. The patient engages a doctor and a handywoman and in some cases the doctor agrees to accept a low fee, it being well understood that he will not be called upon to deliver the patient except in case of emergency. The handywoman manages the labour and the doctor visits the mother on the following day. If nothing goes wrong, it is difficult to prove that the case was not an 'emergency' or a genuine 'born before arrival' or that medical help could have been obtained in time had an effort been made.
>
> It is quite certain that the standard of maternity nursing for the working-class mother will never be raised effectually while these women are allowed to pursue unchecked slipshod, uncleanly methods, especially as many of the poorer women who have never been properly nursed in the past are apt to prefer the homely and time-honoured habits of the handywomen to the methodical routine followed by the careful midwife.[10]

In 1926, the Third Midwives Act banned unqualified people from attending a woman in childbirth unless they could prove that it was a sudden emergency. Again, handywomen and doctors often colluded to find ways around the law.

At a time when many uncertified midwives were being prosecuted and fined for practising midwifery illegally, there does not appear to have been any cases of doctors being prosecuted for their involvement. They were merely warned by their Medical

Council. Undoubtedly, some doctors were responding to the needs of their community by continuing to work with handywomen. However, Mary W., a midwife who worked on the district in a mining town in Yorkshire, is sceptical of their motivation, once certified midwives were in financial competition with doctors:

> A local woman who was capable would attend the birth. They were quite good some of them, bathing the baby and looking after the mother, although they had no idea of sepsis or anything like that. And the doctor would sign all the necessary forms, you see – the birth notifications and that sort of thing. Some of the doctors were very good about the new nurses, but some of them would stick to the handywomen. I had quite a tussle with one of the doctors about employing a handywoman after the 1936 Midwives Act! Because, of course, if there was a handywoman, the doctor would be booked and he would be *paid*. You see, it all boils down to money.

When Mary W. refers to the 'new nurses', she is using the title generally accorded to the new professional midwife who was often at pains to ensure that this was her title, not wanting to be associated with the traditional 'midwife', the handywoman. Katharine L., a midwife who worked on the district in East Anglia, remembers a handywoman who wished to enjoy the status of the title 'nurse':

> There was Mrs A. Now she was one of those kinds of people that everyone would run to, was Mrs. A. There were two or three layers-out in the town too. And then there was Nellie M. – she was a handywoman. And she would often say, 'We *nurses*' if she saw us. I don't know if she used to deliver babies but she went round with the doctors – you know, she might have delivered them, certainly in the days before we came she might well have done. And she would recommend treatment to people and that sort of thing, our Nellie. She was a handywoman, but she thought of herself as a nurse – [laughs] 'We nurses...!'

Nellie M.'s wish to be called 'Nurse' is indicative of the status and power that came with the new title. However, it was not only among practitioners that this was felt. The title, 'midwife' came to be used in a derogatory fashion as the denigration of the handywoman's role permeated through to the people they had traditionally attended. Mollie T., a retired midwifery tutor who comes from a rather privileged background, explains:

> People would refer to the 'odd-job' lady who used to come in and help around the place, as 'the midwife', and the official midwives were known as 'Nurses'. If their patients said, 'Oh, the nurse has been' they meant the midwife. I was always introduced as a nurse and I still find my friends prefer to introduce me in this way. You ask why? I think some of it must go back to Sairey Gamp, the Dickens character – the belief that midwives were dirty, illiterate and drunk – it's very difficult to get rid of that.

It is interesting that nowadays midwives are anxious to make it clear that midwifery is not a branch of nursing. They are often insistent on reclaiming the title, 'midwife' – 'No, I'm not a nurse, I'm a midwife.' The various connotations associated with the titles that midwives choose serve as a reminder of the speed with which midwifery politics have been shifting during this century.

The handywoman was derided as the arch-enemy of midwifery throughout the late 1920s and 1930s, and articles in *Nursing Notes* demonstrate the fervour of the campaign:

> The clause in the Act [Third Midwives Act, 1926] concerning the unqualified person, or handywoman, is only just beginning to be felt, and though it was not as strong as we wished, there is evidence that it can be an efficient *weapon* against the depredations of our *foe* 'the handylady'. [our italics][11]

One midwife[12] described coming across a handywoman who was still attempting to circumvent the law as late as 1945:

> In 1945, I was a pupil midwife doing three months district training in a very poor area of Bristol. On two occasions a handywoman delivered my patients and then sent for Sister and me. Her story was that she happened to look in and the woman was too far on for her to do anything except deliver the baby. On both occasions, the baby had been separated and the placenta expelled.
>
> Sister had met this good lady before, and decided to put an end to her 'help'. She arranged to take her to the M.O.H. [Ministry of Health] so that she herself might notify the birth. I think this frightened her enough to stop any further incidents.

One of the major concerns about the handywoman was that, since she layed out the dead, there was a potentially high risk of her transmitting infection to childbearing women. Ruth Richardson, in her work on handywomen and the laying out of bodies, suggests that throughout the ages, women handed down their skills to their daughters and female relatives.[13] These skills incorporated rituals around handwashing, so the potential dangers of passing infections from corpses to labouring or post-natal women were unwittingly avoided long before sepsis and the transmission of infection were understood. When men became involved in childbirth there was no such tradition of hand-washing, and the soaring rate of deaths due to puerperal sepsis has been well documented.

Early rules of the Central Midwives Board forbade midwives to lay out bodies as a means of trying to prevent the spread of infection, as retired midwifery tutor Mollie T. remembers:

> This thing about laying out bodies was very much in the minds of people in those days. I remember being very aware of the regulations when a neighbour came over to my home and said, 'Mum didn't look so well and could I come over?' Well, Mum was sitting beside the bed and she'd been dead for some considerable time. I explained to them that she was dead – though I didn't say 'for some time' – and could they get the doctor. So they went out to 'phone and came back and said that the doctor had said that if she was dead, there was no point in coming. But this was quite common. I don't think that in the late 1940s many doctors thought there were variations to dying: you were either dead or not. So I retreated, but they came back very shame-faced and said they'd tried to get the woman who did the laying out, but she had 'flu, so would I do it. As I was then working as a general nurse, I went over and did it, but I remember thinking that if this had happened six months earlier when I was working as a midwife, I would have had to have refused because of the CMB regulations that a midwife does not lay out a body except in connection with her practice.
>
> You still hear it being said that midwives in uniform should not mix with nurses. In the days when I was doing nurse training, a sort of caste-system developed in the hospital dining room, where the midwives had to sit at a separate table. This encouraged the belief that they weren't

to be trifled with – and they were quite a savage lot – I wouldn't have trifled with them at all!

But you can understand why there was this ruling. So many women and babies did die from infection in those days...

Maternal mortality

By the 1930s, only a few handywomen continued to flout the law by practising midwifery, and the number of *bona fide* midwives decreased steadily. (The last *bona fide* left the Roll in 1947.) In spite of these developments – and in spite of the advent of antenatal care and the increase in hospital births – the maternal mortality rate rose. From 1924 to 1936, it remained at over five per thousand births.

Few women died at home as a result of childbirth with midwifery care, and as most of the midwives we interviewed worked on the district, their experience of maternal death was limited. In her midwifery textbook, Alice Gregory describes with anguish the devastating effects of a mother dying in childbirth:

> I have twice seen the desolation of a working man's home when the mother is suddenly taken from her young children, and I never want to see it again. She went up to her room in apparently good health perhaps twelve hours before, and she will never come down again until her body is carried to the grave. The little children stand about crying because no one is attending to all their many needs. The father makes an effort with his clumsy hands and abandons it with a gesture of listless despair. A kindly friend probably volunteers to attend to the tiniest of all, but finding that it causes the inevitable gossip among the neighbours, she soon alters her mind, and within a very few months the unhappy man, still aching for the loss of his wife, is forced to put another woman in her place from sheer inability to carry on in any other way. There are few things so absolutely worth doing as the preservation of the life of working mothers – few professions that so satisfy the paramount need of our souls to be of some use to somebody.[14]

Mary W. only saw one mother die in the 37 years that she was a district midwife in Yorkshire, but she still remembers the fear of infection that existed in hospital in an age before antibiotics

were available when over one third of maternal deaths were due
to puerperal fever:

> Yes, the maternal mortality rate was high in the 1930s
> because they had puerperal fever. That was our biggest
> dread – infection. I once saw a septic Caesar while I was in
> Leeds, which was terrible because at Leeds they wouldn't
> do a Caesarean section if they'd even had one vaginal
> examination – they were so terrified of infection. Yes,
> infection was our biggest problem.

Some midwives remembered situations where women were
sent home to have their babies, when hospitals had to be closed
down for 'drastic disinfection' following deaths from puerperal
fever.

In 1924, the first Government Report on Maternal Mortality was
published. This, and subsequent reports on maternal mortality,
highlighted the fact that a large percentage of deaths were
avoidable.

Over the next decade, the issue of maternal mortality was the
focus of much controversy and concern, particularly as it appeared
that as many middle-class as working-class women were dying.
For example, in 1934, deaths from puerperal fever were three times
higher in London's Hampstead, where many women could afford
to be attended by doctors or have their babies in hospital, than
they were in poverty-stricken Bermondsey, where women were
attended by midwives at home.[15]

At a meeting held to debate maternal mortality at Central Hall,
Westminster, on 28 February 1928,[16] it was pointed out that of
all the 'dangerous occupations' in the country, including mining
and seafaring, motherhood was the most dangerous. The deaths
of 3,000 women each year in England and Wales as a result of
child-birth were described as 'a stubborn problem'. It was also
noted that thousands of mothers were unnecessarily damaged or
invalided every year as a result of childbirth, and that the death
rate did not reveal the incalculable loss resulting from unreported
and untreated injury and ill-health arising from pregnancy. The
following resumé of some of the points made at that meeting by
invited speakers – midwives, doctors, members of parliament, dig-
nitaries and social reformers – offers interesting insights into
midwifery politics of the day:

- There is an urgent need to employ more midwives since the midwife more often secures physiological [normal] labour because she is prepared to wait.

- Doctors are 'an expensive social instrument' owing to their long training. It is quite impossible for the doctor to spare the time from his other patients to wait on nature, yet the securing of labour is the basic principle in preventative medicine.

- Maternal morbidity is lowest in those countries with a well-trained corps of midwives, e.g. Holland, Italy and Scandinavian countries. It is highest in the USA, where the services of midwives are not generally or systematically used by the citizens...

- The best trained women do not practice as midwives because though the work is responsible and exacting, the economic return is poor. The future prospects are bad, as 15 years is as long as even the strongest can stand the wear and tear of practice.

- The mothers prefer to be attended by a doctor because such attendance makes possible the use of anaesthesia and the rapid termination of the labour, but for all artificial interference a price has to be paid. The risk in the individual case might be trifling but spread over the country it means a serious increase in the mortality and morbidity rates...

- There is an urgent need for midwives to get more, and regular, post-graduate teaching.

- There is a need to develop National Health Insurance, to develop the work of local authorities in regard to maternity and child welfare, and to improve the general social environment. Expectant mothers should enjoy opportunities of healthy living, healthy homes, and a healthy environment.

- There is a need for more preventative work.

- Although Approved Societies are active in seeing that no person receives a benefit to which he or she is *not* entitled, there is no provision for seeing that all those entitled to benefit receive it... With regard to Maternity there is, of course, the Cash Benefit payable to the insured woman and to the wife of the insured man, but this is swallowed up in payment to doctor or midwife…unless a woman is herself insured, she will have no treatment during pregnancy…

- The Queen Victoria's Jubilee Nurses who work exclusively in the poorest districts have only half the number of maternal deaths that are recorded on an average for England and Wales.

- Research into the causes of maternal mortality should take into consideration the whole circumstances and surrounds of the woman, not only the circumstances of confinement. Maternal mortality and morbidity largely depend on the circumstances of early life and the overall health of the family.

- The Medical Officer of Health can call a midwife before him, and if she has failed in any point he can report her to the Midwives Board. Why can we not do the same with our doctors when they fail?

- There is a need to bring maternity work within the reach of country mothers, including those in very scattered country districts. The first requisite is a good district-nurse-midwife, but the distances they have to cover are far too great and they should be provided with small cars to avoid the waste of strength in bicycling. Motor bicycles are unsuitable as nurses cannot arrive at their case clean and dry.

- Only doctors specially qualified should do antenatal care and no separate payment should be made to doctors for antenatal care under the National Insurance Scheme.

- The Midwives Institute considers that the mother's home is the *safe* place for normal births – antenatal supervision would sift out the abnormal – and if the local authority would spend more money on improving housing rather than building maternity hospitals the maternal mortality would drop.

Although today the maternal mortality rate is less than 0.1 per thousand births, most of the above arguments are as familiar to those involved in the debates surrounding childbirth in the 1990s as they were to the speakers in 1928. However, unlike the recent Health Committee Report on Maternity Services, which advocated a woman-centred approach to childbirth,[17] the most important message to come from the Maternal Mortality Committee Reports of the late 1920s and early 1930s was that the main fault lay with the mothers themselves. Despite evidence showing that 80 per cent of maternal deaths were due to conditions not detectable antenatally – sepsis, haemorrhage and shock – and even though the introduction of antenatal care had proved to be largely ineffective, women were blamed for not making use of what was heralded as the new innovation in preventing maternal deaths:

> There is still a large section of the population that does not realise the advantages of obtaining competent prenatal advice… The patient herself is often her own worst enemy, whether from ignorance or apathy, ill-health or prejudice. Until she is able and willing to co-operate, doctors' and nurses' attempts to assist her can never be fully effective.[18]

The high maternal mortality rates were a major incentive to the government to pass legislation to integrate midwives in private practice within the growing system of public maternity services. The motivation behind the 1936 Midwives Act (*see* Chapter 3) was described in *Nursing Notes*:

> …an all round tightening up as well as strengthening of each link in the chain of obstetric supervision.[19]

During the Second World War changes that contributed to a dramatic decline in maternal deaths were introduced in health care, social services and welfare benefits. The government brought in measures to share available food resources throughout the population, control prices and equalise incomes (*see* Chapter 8). Advances in drugs to counteract infection and control haemorrhage, efficient flying squads (obstetric units that would come from the hospital in an emergency) and blood transfusion services also led to a dramatic decrease in maternal mortality by the end of the war. By 1943 the death rate had fallen to 2.3 per thousand registered births, which was just over half that of the rate in 1935.

The development of a profession

From the First Midwives Act in 1902 to the setting up of the National Health Service in 1948, a succession of developments enforced by statute ensured that eventually the original aim of the Midwives Institute was fulfilled – all women in Britain were entitled to the services of a well-trained corps of midwives (*see*

Appendix 1 – Milestones in Midwifery in Twentieth Century, Pre-NHS Britain).

Whatever we may think about the attitudes and class-ridden tactics of midwifery reformers such as Alice Gregory, who worked to oust the handywomen, there can be no doubt that their actions shaped the foundations of today's profession. Their tireless campaigning, and their manoeuvring within the powerful position accorded to them by society, ensured that midwifery developed as a profession with autonomous practitioner status within a carefully planned legal framework.

It is worth noting than in the various 'colonies' such as the USA, Canada, Australia and New Zealand, where there was often no such opportunity for the campaigners to bend the ear of the 'boys at the top' or to fight the rising tide of capitalist enterprise on the part of doctors, the role of the midwife fast became relegated to the hand-maiden status of the obstetric nurse. In such countries, midwives have had to fight to build or re-build a midwifery profession with the same potential and status as that of the British system.

From our interviews with midwives who worked in Britain in pre-NHS days, it was obvious that they remembered the 1936 Midwives Act as the most significant influence in terms of changes to their working lives, particularly as it implemented a national, salaried midwifery service (*see* chapter 3). However, the women who gave birth at that time tended to describe the setting up of the NHS in 1948 as a turning point in their lives. They described the relief they felt in gaining access to a series of 'free' services, all of which made an enormous impact on the quality of their lives.

The underlying principle of the NHS was that the best of existing health care should be available to every section of the community. It was to be free at the point of service and financed by NHS contributions from those in employment, local rates and central government. While it has been shown that inequalities in health have persisted,[20] there is no doubt that the 1948 Act brought immense relief to many people who were struggling with the consequences of poverty. In the words of Mollie T., who worked as both a nurse and a midwife in the 1940s:

> The Health Service had to come in. People were so poor that they were unable to pay for their care. General patients were coming in too sick for remedial care so it was mostly terminal care, and women weren't getting the care or the

benefits that they needed in pregnancy. But it's taken something away that we haven't yet got back...

Many of the people we interviewed talked wistfully about the passing of an era where birth and death took place mainly in the home, a time when there was plenty of support from neighbours such as the local handywoman.

References

1. Thompson, Flora, *Lark Rise to Candleford*, Penguin Books Ltd, Harmondsworth, UK, 1978, pp.135–136.
2. Gregory, Alice (ed.), *The Midwife: Her Book,* Frowde & Hodder & Stoughton, London, 1923, p.12.
3. *ibid*, p.15.
4. Llewelyn Davies, Margaret (ed.), *Life as We Have Known it – by Co-operative Working Women*, Virago, London, 1977, pp. 43–46, Copyright 1931 Quentin Bell and Angelica Garnett.
5. *Nursing Notes*, March 1905, pp.38–39.
6. *Nursing Notes*, March 1907, pp.42–44.
7. Heagerty, Brooke, *Class, Gender and Professionalization: the Struggle for British Midwifery, 1900–1936*, unpublished dissertation, 1990, Royal College of Midwives' Library.
8. Gregory, Alice (ed.), *op. cit*, p.137.
9. Dickens, Charles, *Martin Chuzzlewit*, Chapman & Hall, London, 1844.
10. Campbell, Janet, *Report on Public Health and Medical Subjects – No.21 The Training of Midwives*, Whitehall, London, June 1923.
11. *Nursing Notes*, January 1928.
12. Letter to the authors from a retired midwife following an appeal in the midwifery press for information about handywomen.
13. Richardson, Ruth, 'Laying Out and Lying In', *Association of Radical Midwives Newsletter*, July 1982, p.4.
14. Gregory, Alice (ed.), *op. cit*, p.135.
15. Roberts, Dr. Harry, 'The Price of Motherhood', *The News Chronicle*, 14 May 1934.
16. *Maternal Mortality – Report of Meeting Held at Central Hall, Westminster, on February 28th 1928*, published by The Maternal Mortality Committee, 1928.

17. *House of Commons Health Committee Report on Maternity Services*, HMSO, London,1992.
18. *Departmental Committee on Maternal Mortality and Morbidity*, 1930, pp.24–25, 39.
19. Quoted in 'Maternal Mortality', Memorandum 156/MCW, *Nursing Notes*, January 1931, p.4.
20. Townsend, Peter and Davidson, Nick, *Inequalities in Health – The Black Report & The Health Divide*, Penguin Books, London, 1990.

2 Handywomen: 'the woman you called for'

> She saw you into the world and she saw you out the other end… It was just the thing that you called for her.

The title 'handywoman' presumably developed as a description of the many tasks that might be carried out by 'the woman you called for'. Our research confirms previous findings that the primary role of the handywoman before she was ousted in the early part of the century was that of midwife. Most handywomen also laid out the dead.[1]

Molly B. and her sister, Lily N., grew up in South Shields, Tyneside, in the 1920s. They have vivid memories of Granny Anderson, their 'midwife', and the important role she played within the local community. Their descriptions of her paint a picture far removed from the 'dirty, garrulous, drink-sodden, Sairey Gamp' image that was constantly levelled at the old midwives by those who saw them as the perpetrators of infection and dangerous practice:

> *Lily:* Mum was 17 when she married in 1914. She had eight children altogether and every one of them was brought into the world at home by Granny Anderson, this woman down the road that had no medical qualifications whatsoever. Every time anybody was having a baby, you used to see them running down the back lane for Granny Anderson. She always came and bathed the babies and that; followed the babies up. You weren't allowed to put your feet out of bed for two weeks in those days.

> *Molly:* She was quite plump and all in black. And she wore – I don't know if you've ever seen them – one of those little black bonnets, a bit like Queen Victoria used to wear. All in black, but she always had a pure white apron on. And

she actually turned it up at the corners and tucked it into
her belt to keep the inside clean till she got to you. And
always a black shawl. Very few women up in the North at
that time had a coat – they all used to wear shawls tied
round the shoulders. She had a beaded black bag over her
arm – like a shopping bag with two handles.

Lily: I never knew if she was a widow. I never saw a man
there and I went to her house several times. She didn't have
children as far as I knew. She seemed to be completely on
her own. I never heard her first name. Even the doctor called
her Granny Anderson. She was quite a matriarch. Everyone
was quite fearful of Granny Anderson. But everyone used
her in the road.

Molly: Ooh yes, she was very abrupt. We was quite
frightened of her really. I mean, if your mother sent you
for Granny Anderson, you used to run like the clappers up
the back lane to get to her. And your house had to be
spotlessly clean before she'd enter. Scrubbed out with
carbolic. D'you remember? – No, you wouldn't know the
carbolic soap. It was white and blue, a marbley thing and
it was horrible actually. But everything was scrubbed out
before a birth with carbolic. She used to give you a list of
what had to be ready or to hand, like torn sheets, piles of
newspapers and boiling water – because nobody had
running water. There was a tap in the yard and a range that
you cooked on. We used to have to save the newspapers for
her and she'd spread it out around and on the bed. And then
torn sheets for draw sheets and pads.

Lily: Yes, she got the house scrubbed out with carbolic
and there was always a bowl of hot water and carbolic
soap for Granny Anderson to wash her hands in – that was
one of the musts. I can remember seeing her scrubbing her
hands. The kitchen table was always laid out and, of course,
they always scrubbed the kitchen table.

Molly: If you were misbehaving outside she'd tell you. I think
she was more for women than she was for men, you know.
She just dismissed the men as 'OUT!'... You know, 'You're
a useless sort of bunch of people'...instead of encouraging
them to be there (and they might have changed their
mind a bit about sex then if they'd been there). But she sort
of shooed them out of the place. She would never allow the

men there, would she? They would be completely banished. They were of no use to Granny Anderson.

Mum said Granny Anderson was furious with dad when I was born. I weighed three and a half pounds and she'd been in labour 24 hours and he said when they showed him me, he said 'God, all that fuss over *that*!' And Granny Anderson was furious with him. Oh yes, he was banished because of his remarks!

Lily: She used to lay out the bodies, too, and you always had a drawer in those days. The old people used to have a bottom drawer and all their laying out stuff would be in it – ready for you to be laid out for when you died.

Molly: Yes, she laid out Aunty Kitty and all the babies and that. I remember Aunty Jane's little Georgina dying because of course they had the coffin in the bedroom – they had nowhere else to put it. It was either in the living room where you had all your meals and that or in the bedroom.

Granny Anderson may not have been a qualified professional, but she knew how to cope with most situations. She liaised with the local doctor and people referred to her for advice about illnesses at a time when the doctor's fees were prohibitive:

Lily: All the babies were born at home. Our mum had some funny births. John was four pounds, first baby, and she was ill in bed for three months after that through haemorrhaging. I think that time Granny Anderson actually called the doctor. They thought she was going to have twins but it turned out to be only one child. You were born with your arm coming out first and weighed three and a half pounds and one of them was born with the caul on.

Molly: Granny Anderson was very capable. Most people used to go to her for illnesses, too. The doctor referred people to her but I don't think he worked with her because no-one had the money to pay him. She used to do minor ailments, like sore throats. One of them for sore throats was half an onion, covered in brown sugar. They still do it, some people actually, don't they? You cut and sliced the onion, put brown sugar on it and then put a basin on it and when it sort of melted and the juice ran out, you just spooned that in for sore throats and colds. That cough mixture you get now, Liquifruta, that's made of sort of the same stuff.

Neither of the sisters could remember seeing any financial transactions take place around Granny Anderson and they thought that she was paid in kind – 'People gave her things'. They were clearly horrified at the suggestion that she might have been paid with 'a tot of rum':

> *Lily*: Goodness, no. I'm sure she was never paid with a tot of rum. In fact, I can't remember any women up there ever drinking. They weren't allowed in the pubs any rate in those days – well, they might have been down by the river with all the sailors coming in but not where we were. I never remember any woman going into a pub. At Christmas, I think they might have had a bottle of port and everyone had a little drink, but that was it.

It was hard for Molly and Lily to imagine that anyone could take the place of Granny Anderson in the community:

> *Molly*: She must have died somewhere around the beginning of the war when we'd all moved away and completely lost touch. When we came back Granny Anderson was no longer around but she would have carried on practising right until she died. Yes, even though you say it wasn't legal. Up there lots of people did things that wasn't legal. Granny was still doing her rounds years and years after we were grown up and moved away.

Reports written in the first decades of this century paint a picture of the untrained midwife that is rather different from the efficient, carbolic-loving Granny Anderson remembered by Molly and Lily:

> As long as she [the handywoman] undertakes any form of nursing or personal care of the mother, she is a potential danger, and the more she knows the more dangerous she is because she is tempted to interfere, or even act as a midwife. She has no recognised qualification or position, she is under no jurisdiction or authority, she can defy all the rules which a midwife must observe and her dirty fingers must be responsible for a large amount of minor and major sepsis. [Whitehall 1923][2]

There is, in fact, no evidence to suggest that handywomen were in any major way dealing out 'death and destruction' or that they were involved in providing abortions – another accusation levelled at them. Written accounts of the day, plus the testimony that we gathered, suggest that individual handywomen varied as much as individual midwives in terms of whether people saw them as 'good' or 'bad'. Most of the women we interviewed who spoke harshly about handywomen were describing what Edie M. called 'dodgy looking after' rather than life-threatening practice:

> Twice I was unlucky with the woman I got in. It all depends on who you get, how well you get looked after. If you were unlucky, then you wouldn't get cooked for, your washing done and all that. If they only came in for an hour or so in between looking after their own family, you never got much. I never got a woman that gave me a lot of care. As I say, Mrs. M. was a close friend – the daughter went into films with Monty Banks – she was a close friend but she used to come in full of poverty...starving hungry, saying, "Ain't had a bit in my lips today, Edie'. I'd say, 'Well, put kettle on and go round the corner and get some cakes – twelve for sixpence'. The dairy used to make them out of their cracked eggs – so on would go the kettle. Oh, I had some dodgy looking after. But you didn't pay them much for the ten days, there wasn't a lot of money about.

Lou N. was one of several other women who remembered being attended by rather 'needy' or acquisitive handywomen:

> I had the midwife there, the woman that came in, but she made herself so much at home. 'Oooh, I like this, I like that', and it ended up – you were giving her more than what she did! She took a fancy to my macintosh and she went on and on till she got this macintosh off me. She was a midwife, a local woman; there was nothing professional about her.

Ruby C. was also unimpressed with the handywoman who attended her when she had her second baby in Ireland:

> When Maureen was born, I had to have a doctor then 'cause there was no nurse in the village. And an old lady of 70 came. Oh God, she nearly drove me crackers! And d'you know what she did with our Maureen? She believed in bringing a baby up hardy, you know, in the country way. Maureen was born on the sixth of December. We had a big barrel of rain water outside and she brought in a bath from it! She had to break the ice on the water! [laughs] So our Maureen should have been tough!

In those days you had to lie in bed ten days. And you mustn't get out, mustn't do anything, you know, hardly get out to the toilet, and anyway, as soon as she'd gone home I used to jump out of bed and dust all around the bedroom, y'know and tidy it up, 'cause the way she'd done it didn't please me. [laughs] It's laughable in a way, but it wasn't funny at the time. She was a proper old countrywoman.

The next one I had, by then they'd gone in for training and so I had this nurse and she delivered the baby and everything. She was very good – just as good as a doctor, like.

Jane W. remembers her first birth experience as being 'fairly ghastly' due to conflict with the handywoman. In literature and testimony we came across several references to handywomen encouraging women to 'bear down' before they were ready – a disadvantageous practice that could exhaust the mother and expose the baby to a certain amount of risk:

I'd booked up with the Medical Mission because them times I was a bit nervous of men doctors, and they had a lady doctor there. They asked me to book up with them. Before that I'd engaged a woman. My cousin, she'd just had a baby and she was all right the next day after it. So I thought that the woman must be good, and I asked her if I could have her woman to look after me, which I did. I engaged her.

Anyway, I'd been out the day before with one of me sisters, walked miles we had. Used to be a great walker. So I came home and there was me landlady waiting for me. She says, 'The nurse has been here from the Medical Mission and she's left these pills. You've got to take one every hour, and a large dose of castor oil, and then when the pains start, send for the doctor'. Oh dear! I didn't know where I was. I'd had no experience or nothing, didn't know what to do!

So anyway, I did it all and I started – you know – didn't know if it was the castor oil, whether it was the baby, what was happening to me. So I thought I'd best send for that woman first. My husband went and got the woman, and my eldest sister came round and stayed with me. This woman, she smelt of drink, she wasn't my type at all, not nice at all. [laughs] She was telling me what to do. And meanwhile my husband got all the pennies and filled the meter up – it was gas, we had no electricity. Of course, they was making cups of tea and all that, getting ready.

So anyway, the pains got more regular and then I sent and told the doctor. The doctor and the nurse arrived. The doctor said, 'Oh, my dear. It's nowhere near ready yet. You want *rest*'. Don't do this, don't do that – all the things the woman had been telling me to do. She'd been telling me to bear down whenever I got a pain. She'd got a towel and folded it and I had to grasp it. She'd fixed it over the top of the bed – 'Get on the bed, pull it and bear down.'

Anyway, the doctor stopped all that, so of course the woman got a bit nasty. She said, '*I'm* supposed to see to her'. She did no more. The doctor turned the woman out. She said, 'Don't you come in this room again. '*I'm* in authority'. And she turned her out. So anyway, every now and then she'd try to come back in and she was pushed out. A little tiny nurse was with the doctor and it was all back pains with me. I'd say, 'Oh, me back, me back'. And this little nurse would rub me back. She was very good.

Well, anyway, it went on hour after hour. And then early in the morning, I was wishing I was dead and all the rest of it. And in the end the baby did arrive. I don't know, I was half demented with pain because he was a big baby – 9lbs 4ozs. And I was small, small-built inside. And he tore me badly. The doctor started to see to me, to stitch me up. The worst that could happen – the gas ran out – total darkness, no more gas. She had a torch with her so she had to finish stitching me up by torch.

So then my husband paid the woman off and told her not to come back tomorrow. We'd manage without her. But she was a terrible experience, she was. And she smelt of drink. I still don't like drink.

Mrs G's gems

I'd get called all times of the night and day. It was either to get one in or to take one out.

It is rare to find a handywoman alive. Most were mature women when they were practising in the first decades of this century. Mrs G. was 95 years old when we interviewed her in 1989. She was the ninth of 18 children and was a handywoman in the London Borough of Bexleyheath for 50 years. She described being seen as something of an expert since the age of 13, when she delivered

a baby for the first time. This was presumably under the supervision of her mother, who was a midwife. It would have been interesting to find out more about Mrs G.'s mother – particularly
how she managed to get training and work as an employed
midwife as well as rear 18 children. Unfortunately, Mrs G. would
not be drawn into giving more than a few tantalising comments:

> My mother was a midwife for 50 years. Some of the time
> she was paid by the East End Council. My mother was
> trained. She trained at Stourbridge Hospital 'cause they
> used to live up that way. Then she went to the London
> Hospital and then she went to a hospital, in the Midlands.
> She had a proper tuition, she did. [proudly]
>
> Oh yes, she had to pay for her tuition. You didn't get your
> jam for nothing. You had to buy everything then. They're
> lucky these days, though I don't think the training's so
> severe as it was. Good job really for the nurses' sake.
>
> She taught me a lot about midwifery. I don't think you
> can beat it really. It's nice to be able to bring another life
> into the world. But some little mites are so deformed and
> terrible. It's nice to know we're not all perfect isn't it? I say,
> if a baby's born healthy and perfect, that's all you want. You
> can bring it up properly then. That's right.
>
> My mother said, 'Never be frightened. Whatever comes,
> never be frightened'.
>
> When the war was on my mother was very old then. She
> went to the church when the church was bombed. My
> mother crawled under the stone and all that and delivered
> a baby boy. She said, 'I'm going to get that baby out.
> There's a mother crying in there about having a baby and
> I'm going in there to get it out'. A 9lb baby boy. Of course
> they had to go to hospital but they was both all right.
> Marvellous isn't it!
>
> Oh no, she wasn't *my* midwife. You mustn't mix pork and
> beef – never. No...[confused] pork with pork [contradict-
> ing herself]... The last baby I delivered was Sandra, my
> granddaughter. House opposite. I delivered two of my
> grandchildren. Oh yes, I believe in keeping it in the family.

Any romantic ideas we might have had about handywomen
were quashed by Mrs G's accounts of how she supported women
and their families during labour, all of which were interspersed
with hearty laughter:

Some say, 'Oh never mind dear, never mind. That's no good at all'. You have to say, 'Come along. 'Course you can get it out. 'Course you can. Don't be stupid. I'll put your head in a bucket of water if you don't shut up!' They used to laugh. It used to pass the time, you see. It's the only way to keep them cheerful. 'Cause of course, some people are terrified. I think it's other people talking to them before the baby's actually going to be born, they frighten them you see and that's it.

Now fancy a midwife, when the woman's crying with the pain, she's sitting there, wiping her own tears! That's stupid! I used to say to them, 'You're not ready for the asylum yet mate! Shut up!' I'd say, 'Any more of this and I'm gonna leave yer! Get on with it'. 'Oh no, you won't, will you?' and I'd say, 'Won't I? Just you try me.' And I'd say, 'You've 'ad yer sweets, now you must 'ave yer sours...'

I used to tell the fathers to do what they were told and all. I used to say to the father sometimes, you know, 'You mind your business now. You've had your share!'

No, the fathers were never there at the birth, never, no. I don't know, maybe he should be? If he puts it there, why can't he see it come out?... see the work he's done, all the trouble he's caused? That's true, isn't it? I dunno...but still, there you are...

I wouldn't say people helped each other out more, no. I'd say they just got on with it. You have to get on with it, don't you? You don't not make a fuss when it's put there and then make a damn fuss when it comes away. Goes in a little bit and it comes out a damn great lump!

The children were never there [at the births], no. I didn't like it if there were children about. If the mother left it too late and there was no one to take the children, I used to say to them, 'Clear off, I've cut me finger'. They'd say, 'All that blood comes from your finger?...' And I'd say, 'Yes. Buzz off!' [laughter] They used to look at me, sweet like. You don't know what to say for the best, do you? You can't open their eyes too much though, can you? They used to laugh at me though, some of them.

In Chapter 11, we can see that although Mrs G's understanding of the anatomy and physiology of childbirth was decidedly limited and her practice at times somewhat meddlesome, nothing she described could be labelled as 'dangerous' or 'life threatening'. Mrs G. was proud of having received a double award for first-aid

from the St. John's Ambulance Service and the Red Cross. People
obviously saw her as an expert to whom they could turn in a
variety of situations:

> When people were sick, I used to go and sit with them at
> night. Or if they were a bit barmy I used to go with them.
> What's the good of being frightened of people?
>
> One lad, who's sailed round the world, when he was little,
> his mother brought him to me. She said, 'I spilled soup on
> him.' I said, 'Good! [laughs] All right bring him in'. So I sat
> him up on the table, cut the back of his shoe off, got it off
> and done it up. And I said, 'It's not hurting, is it, love?' 'No,
> it's not hurting'. So I said, 'That's all right then'. I said, 'Bring
> him back tomorrow morning and don't you touch it'. 'All
> right', she said. So she brought him back every morning for
> a week. Anyway I got it better for him and he was all right
> and happy with it. And every time he saw me as he grew
> up, he said, 'My foot's still better!' I'd say, 'You're asking
> for trouble, boy!' [laughs] Oh, there's been some funny
> people in this road... Never mind!

A different sort of handywoman

> She would go into any old 'pig-sty' and not bat an eye-lid.

When people talked about 'the woman you called for', they
referred to a local, working-class woman. However, midwife
Mollie T. remembered 'somebody who would go' who came from
a very different background:

> When I was young, we lived in a small village on the Kent
> coast. In about 1935, we moved away, but I used to go back
> every year to stay with an elderly lady and her husband. She
> was quite an interesting person because she was the niece
> of William Rathbone, who started all the health care in
> Liverpool, and as a family they were very public-spirited.
> She must have been quite a threat in the village, but the
> Jubilee [a trained midwife; *see* Chapter 3] seemed to get on
> very well with her and I'm sure she had an unofficial
> liaison with her. I'm sure they worked together quite a bit,
> but nobody was supposed to know about it.
>
> When I was staying there, there was an emergency call
> to a cottage in the next village. When we got up there, the
> woman had had her baby unattended, and I gathered from

noises off that she was bleeding quite considerably, but I didn't get told anything.

There were quite a lot of children around in a very small space and it was very squalid. I was quite confused, but I was set to work, washing up and getting the kids washed, while this old family friend of ours got going. Having dealt with everything she then sent a message to the Jubilee midwife, who said that if she was there, it was OK and she'd come up the next day.

I think quite a lot of this sort of thing did go on. It was bound to when you had a single-handed person out in the country with no transport besides her own two feet. This old family friend had had no training but everyone knew that she would turn a hand to anything that needed doing; that she would go into any old 'pig-sty' and not bat an eyelid, and work untramelled through the most awful conditions. But she had no official capacity at all. She was just 'somebody who would go'.

Laying-out

The dead can't hurt you. I've laid out hundreds.

Handywoman Mrs G. was eager to talk about her role as the person who was called to lay out the dead and to describe the intricacies of this task. Although she was unforthcoming as to whether people paid her for midwifery work (possibly because of its illegal status), laying-out was definitely a task for which she was paid:

Yes, of course they used to pay me for the laying out. Well, some people did. If they were dead I laid them out, 'course I did. The dead can't hurt you. I've laid out hundreds. I'd get called all times of the night and day. It was either to get one in or to take one out.

I laid out my mother's grandmother. No, my mother didn't teach me. I laid out my first body on my own. My mother said that was the best way to learn. But I used to go with my mother sometimes to lay out bodies. It's no trouble laying a body out. As I say, you live and learn, love, as you go through life. You can't expect to learn everything at once. You've got to learn gradually.

It's nothing to be frightened of. People say, 'Ooh, it must be difficult', but it's not. It's easy. They used to say,

'How do you wash them?' And I would say, 'With soap and water, mate!'

It would frighten the death out of people, and I'd say, 'What did you cover their face for, stupid?' I never cover dead persons' faces. Why should you? They're not doing you any harm. They can't pull faces at you, can they?! Why worry?

So you'd wash them and make them look nice. You'd wash their face naturally, then their front, put a towel on the bed, turn them over and wash their back, and then if it's a man you'd get a shirt – if he's an awkward size and you can't get it on him, you'd have to slit it up the back, then slip it over their arms, you see, and then just draw it with linen thread through the middle. It's so simple when you know how. It was no trouble.

I used to wash them all over and then put a clean shirt or a clean nightdress on and a clean pillow-case and sheet. But when I laid them out I always used to leave one hand out of the bedclothes, and I would put a Bible or a flower in their hand. That's how I would do it so they would look natural. But some people didn't. Some people, when they lay out a body, they do the silliest thing. They put the arms across it. Stupid thing to do 'cause sometimes the undertaker has to break them to get them down [in the coffin], you see.

One thing they nearly always do, nearly everyone passes a death motion. They nearly always do, so I used to get a napkin or an old towel and pass it through like a nappy. Then, if they done anything, there's nothing for the undertaker to get his hands in or anything. You have to think of all these things. It's amazing what there is to be taught in life, really. There is an easy way and there's a hard way.

And a clean sheet over them, but never over their chin, always under the chin. I used to comb their hair and make it look nice, and of course, push their jaw up. You have to do that and you have to hold the eyes down for a while, pennies on the eyes. Then you just put a bit of cotton wool inside them for a few minutes. If the jaw won't stop up, you get a bit of bandage and you tie it round onto their head while you wash another part of the body. Then, when you've finished, you just take it off 'cause by then it's set. D'you know what I mean?

When I finish, they say, 'Don't they look nice. Are they asleep?' I say, 'Yes, they're having a good sleep now'. I say, 'No good you looking at them now. They won't talk now. Come on'. And away they go.

I'll tell you a funny story. A man lived down the road here. He thought he was a gentleman. He thought he was, but he wasn't. And his sister died. Died on Christmas morning. I had my granddaughter there and she was playing, 'Show Me the Way to go Home' on the piano. When I opened the door, he was on the step crying. He said, 'Guess who's gone?' And I said, 'Where've they gone to?' So he said, 'She died', and I said, 'Don't talk rubbish'. He said, 'She's dead. Will you come down?' I said, 'Yes, I'll come'. So I went down, away I went down.

I had to get her nightdress off to do that job. You have to cut it up the back. So I did that. Then I tidied her up as best I could after I'd washed her. Then I wrapped the nightie up in newspaper and took it down to the daughter-in-law and asked her to burn it. She said, 'What is it?' I said, 'You mind your own business. Just burn it please'. It was the nightdress and you didn't want that lying about.

So the next day, he comes up and he says, 'What did you do with her nightdress?' And I says, 'You ask her daughter-in-law, she burned it'. And he says, 'What, a *new* nightdress?!' [laughter] Fancy coming and asking for it – a man – what's he want a nightdress for?!

So, he said, 'I'll give you one of them souvenirs from Jessie because you know she thought a lot of you'. I said, 'I don't want it'. So he said, 'Will you come down to my house?' So I said, 'Yes, I'm not frightened of you'.

So, he said, 'Come upstairs'. So I went upstairs and he had a little cupboard by the fireplace. So he said, 'Now I've got some nice things for you here'. And he pulled out an old pair of corsets, one of them that laces up the back! So he says, 'A lovely pair of corsets here'. So I said, 'What will I do with them? I don't wear them!' I said, '*You* wear them! The damn dirty things!' They'd been quite good once but not any more! He must have been quite mad. I said to him, 'I'm not taking that dirt out of your home and into mine. Not likely!'

He comes to visit me sometimes and he still talks about me refusing the corsets! But if you heard him, you'd think he was a gentleman! [mimics accent]

Mrs G. had many other stories about laying out the dead but she referred to this one as her favourite:

> I'm going to tell you a joke. You won't never believe it! Now when I was about 24 or 25 I was staying with my sister and the man next door to her he died. At half eight one evening, the wife came along and she said, 'Can you come? There's something the matter with Jimmy. I don't know what it is. I couldn't tell you 'cause I've run away'. So I went in and I went upstairs and I said, 'I'm sorry, I can't help him now 'cause he's dead, y'see'.
>
> I had to wait for a doctor to come and certify the death before I could move him. So the doctor came and gave me the registration of the dead – 'cause the undertaker won't come until you've got that.
>
> His wife wanted him brought down and put in the front room on the table. They used to do that one time. Well, the funny part is, he was rather a tall man, and anyway I got him along the passage and onto the landing – I put him on a blanket and pulled him along by myself, dead. By myself, I was. I was it all. Funny thing though was, I couldn't get him down the stairs. So I walked past him on the landing like, and there was two men come by the front door of the house, so I said, 'Excuse me, would you be kind enough to come and give me a help?' They said, 'Yes, Madam, certainly we will.'
>
> Well, there was this dead bloke on the stairs but I'd got a blanket under him so we could pull him on that. So I said, 'I'll take his shoulders'. That meant I had to bend over him. 'You two men, you take the weight from his torso to his feet. Go each side of him and one take one leg and one take the other, but put your hand up his back so his back don't break.' Though it wouldn't have mattered 'cause he's dead!
>
> Anyway, 'I think we'll manage', I said. And these two men, they stood each side of him but of course the staircase is not very wide. I think we got him down about three stairs after that, maybe about half way down, and of course moving the body caused it to let out wind! And what happened? These two men, they dropped him and they ran!
>
> They left me and as they dropped him, I fell over and was laying on top of him and d'you know, he wouldn't make love to me at all!
>
> I got him down in the end and got him into the front room. Then I took one of the panels out of the table, put

it down like that, put the blanket on it, then him on the blanket, then I went to the other side of the table, pulled the blanket and sort of levered him up onto the table. Then I said, 'You're all right now, matey!'

And my arm and my chest was aching with the weight of it. But fancy two men running away!

Many handywomen, like Mrs G., found that laying out became the main focus of their work once legislation made it impossible for them to practise as midwives. Over the next decades, however, death, like birth, became progressively more institutionalised. Today, most people will be laid out in a hospital or in the premises of an undertaker. The chances are that the last rites will be performed by a stranger rather than by a neighbour, relative or friend.

Resistance to the new midwives

You see, they thought that experience counted more than training...

While the handywoman tended to be an older woman known to everyone by name, the new, certified midwife was likely to be young, middle-class and wearing a uniform, the official badge of her status and training. From the testimony we gathered, it appears that the relationships between professional midwives and their clients were sometimes acrimonious when there was a recent memory of a handywoman losing her livelihood due to the new legislation. Elizabeth C., who worked in Battersea, describes the resistance she encountered on the district in the 1930s:

The handywomen were illegal then, you see. You had some who were very jealous of your being there to do it because they'd always done it. You'd meet those ones, the ones that were really upset – you know, they'd do things like they wouldn't give you hardly any boiling water. I remember one superintendent [on a supervisory visit] saying, 'You haven't got much water, Miss C.?' I said, 'Well, I can't get it. I've tried everything. Her father and all the people around her are resistant'. The father's mother, or someone, used to do it, you see. So I couldn't get anything out of them. I just had the bare necessity out of them and no more.

It must have been hard for them when they couldn't practise anymore because it was their livelihood, not that it was much of a livelihood for them. They didn't get much apparently, but then people didn't have much.

Mary W., who grew up in a Yorkshire mining town, experienced resistance to change of a different sort when she returned to the area to work as a qualified midwife in the 1930s:

> The image of the midwife was of a mature, motherly old lady, and I didn't get on at all well to begin with. I remember having quite a battle with one of my old aunts. She came and watched me bath this baby and she said, 'I like flannels on bairns'. 'Oh', I said, 'Well, I do occasionally but there's no need for it'. And, of course, my new ideas took a lot of getting used to with these people, and it was quite a fight with the grandmothers. You see, in a village, these old customs are hard to eliminate. 'Me grandma says this and me grandma says that!'
>
> They had some very peculiar old remedies. I once went to a house and this woman had a breast abscess. This was something you very often got because of the lack of antibiotics. And she said, 'Me mother-in-law's put me a cow clap poultice on today'. Oh dear! Can you imagine? Cow dung on an open abscess! They had great faith in cow dung poultices! And this old woman – oh, she was a frightful old thing! So I put a stop to that very quickly and told the old lady off. You had to fight them.
>
> And putting the babies in bed with them, that was another thing you had to fight. They sometimes had a cradle that was passed down through the family, and some of them wouldn't mind using a drawer or something to put the baby in if they didn't have a cot. But then again, you'd usually go and find the baby in bed with its mother, you know. And strangely enough, there were very few cot deaths in those days!... [*see* Chapter 11]

When we suggested to Mary W. that women might have accepted her because she was a local woman who had married and had a baby herself, she retorted:

> Married with a baby, yes. But coming from round here, *no*. Because – have you heard the expression – 'A rabbit isn't a rabbit in his own country?'

Once I was really hurt. A woman I'd known all my life, and she said to someone, 'I can't see how she knows so much. She's no' but a lass!' And I was 25 then and done four years in hospital, besides doing midwifery training! So I was really quite hurt about it. I think of course you think 'I'm going to show them'. But, you see, they thought that experience meant more than training...

Handywomen and midwives working together

There was women that followed Elsie and did the donkey work for her... The family paid these women.

In the late 1930s, legislation had ensured that all local councils were providing a midwifery service. By this time, the role of the handywoman had changed almost beyond recognition. She was no longer 'the midwife'. Instead, she had become the 'odd-job woman' or 'the woman who does' – often working alongside the midwife. Mary T., who lived for most of her life with Elsie Walkerdine, a certified midwife, explained to us how women in Deptford, south-east London, employed a handywoman to work alongside Elsie:

There was always a women that followed Elsie and did the donkey work. She used to take home the washing and the mother's dirty linen and such like, and she used to turn round and get a meal for them if they had other children and there was no one else.

Oh, Elsie very, very seldom had to do her own donkey work. The family paid these women. At the births they did the donkey work, got the water, cleared up, looked after the other kids – all that sort of thing.

Sissy S. had several babies with Elsie Walkerdine as the midwife in attendance. Here, she describes the working relationship between Elsie Walkerdine and the various handywomen. It is a relationship not unlike the much-praised Dutch system today, where the maternity-aid nurse works alongside the midwife, carrying out practical tasks at home births and in the postnatal period:

There would be the lady there to get the hot water, soap, flannels and towels, and she'd wait on Nurse Walkerdine. She was like Nurse Walkerdine's assistant. She was always there before Nurse Walkerdine got there. When you was in

labour you sent for Mrs P. She would be there – 'Have you
sent for Nurse?' – 'Yes, Mr S. has just gone round'. 'Oh good,
I'll get the kettles on.' And she had everything ready. I mean,
us automatically got our bits and pieces together in a
drawer, what we had to have, but Mrs P. would get all the
hot water and wait on Nurse Walkerdine. And when she was
finished, 'D'you want a cup of coffee or tea, nurse?' 'No, I
won't stop because I'm expecting another call...' or
sometimes she would stop.

Mrs P. would stay on, tidy up, do the washing and see
to the other children, and then at dinner time she'd go
home, but she'd come back at night after their dad had
given them tea to make sure they'd had a wash, or to put
them to bed. And that was £2 – £2 with a pint of beer every
night! We paid the midwife £2 and the woman what did
£2. At that time my husband used to earn £2.10s a week,
so you saved up your sixpences. That £2 for the midwife
covered her ten days of visiting, and Mrs P. would also come
for the ten days.

Esther S., who lived and worked as a midwife in the area of
Portsmouth in which she grew up, paid tribute to a handywoman
known affectionately in the community as Ma Sturgess:

The handywoman is part of some of my earliest memories
of my midwifery life. In that area of Portsmouth, everyone
knew each other very well and there was a woman called
Ma Sturgess – everybody called her Ma or Ma Sturgess.
She was very ordinary, very homely, hair screwed back
and up in a bun – a typical 'Ma' that one would think of
as a Ma. And she took the role of, well, if anyone needed
any help in any way, she was the one that would go.

She would be called to lay out the dead and she'd go in
for the sick as well. Sometimes she'd sit up all night. We all
just sort of sent for Ma – maybe that's why she was known
as Ma.

I expect they paid her in kind because she had five
children to bring up on her own. She was a widow. But she
didn't do it for that reason. She wasn't like a paid person
in any official capacity. It was just word-of-mouth and
kindness.

Of course, I knew her because she was the mother of
children that I'd been at school with. (Like me, her children
would have been born in the 1910s.) She was so well-

known that if anything went wrong up the school, Ma Sturgess was up there! [laughter] – 'Ooh, she's up the school again, Ma Sturgess!' – she was a person that never let anything die! A very strong woman, a real character.

Her niece came down from London to stay to have her baby and I delivered her niece in Ma's house. And we had twins! – Margaret and George. They were the only set I had that were boy/girl and I had seven sets of twins on the community. And of course the niece had to go back to London with them but that will tell you how well thought of she was.

She was, as you would say, a most useful person. I'd go into a home and invariably Ma would be there, getting things ready, getting the water on. I might be out on another call, and she'd wait with the patient. She would calm them, make a cup of tea, be friendly with them. She'd say, 'You'll be all right by the time nurse comes...' That sort of thing. She was 'handy' inasmuch as she did that part. But I have known situations where I've been extremely busy, and I've been called out literally when I'd just had a delivery. I'd have got the mother and the baby straight – and she'd say, 'Well, that's all right, you leave them to me, nurse. Everything's all right, you've done the cord and everything...' She knew what to do. She knew it all, you bet, inasmuch as I could go off to another delivery and then I would go back later. I mean, she was a person that you knew you could trust and the mums were in very good hands.

With Ma, my confidence in her was such that I never worried that she'd do anything other than be there to *assist*. I mean, the trust was such that she didn't hang on to send for you. She just sent for you when she got there. Meanwhile, she started getting everything organised. We had a very good working relationship, Ma and I.

I do remember my mother used to talk to me about her mother and she was a similar sort of person – everyone went to her in the village [in Dorset] and they used to call her 'Granny Bolt Upright' because she was so tall and slim! Yes, *she* was the person that everybody always went to. My mother was one of ten children and she always used to tell me about her mother – Granny Bolt Upright.

After the National Health Service was set up in 1948, the role of 'the woman that you called for' diminished further. With an organised, state-funded home help service and increasing hospi-

talisation for both birth and death, the handywoman faded into
extinction.

A tribute to Alice W.: 'the woman you called for'

> My mother was this little Geordie woman and she was a
> fighter you see...

When Ken W. offered to talk to us about his mother, who was a
handywoman, he was insistent that his sister, Florence, would be
able to offer a better interview – partly because she was older and
her memory would stretch back further and partly because she had
trained as a midwife with the Salvation Army. Interestingly, this
was not to be the case.

While acknowledging that her mother was 'a marvellous mother
who was always there for us children', Florence was resistant to
talking about her mother's work as a handywoman. She gave the
impression that years of conditioning in a system that poured scorn
on 'the old Gamps' had lead her to feel that there was something
shameful about the role of the handywoman, that such topics were
best forgotten.

Ken, on the other hand, related vivid memories that placed his
mother's work within the wider context of her life and struggle
for existence. This chapter therefore, ends with a tribute to the life
and work of Alice W., as remembered by her son, Ken, who died
in 1991:

> My mother was born in 1884, in Shotley Bridge, near
> South Shields, and her mother died in childbirth. Her
> father had been a regular army man in the Artillery when
> they had cannon guns, and he got deaf because he got his
> eardrums shattered, and so they got him a job as a level
> crossing keeper at Shotley Bridge. And he got killed by a
> train because he couldn't hear! She'd been living with her
> dad at the level crossing, so there she was, an orphan at 14.
> So she was made a ward of court to her uncle. She ran away
> from him when she was 16 to an auntie and uncle in
> South Walsham in Suffolk. The auntie was the village
> nurse and the uncle the village schoolteacher.
> They got her a job in the fever hospital in Great Yarmouth
> when fever hospitals were very big institutions, especially
> in a sea port. They asked for volunteers to go nursing

there, and she did. And evidently they had a smallpox outbreak and that's where she met my father.

She had 13 children and I found out recently from my sister, Florence, that she had several miscarriages as well. I don't think in the particular culture of Yarmouth in that time it was very remarkable – they all had lots of children. I was number twelve and there must have been more than 20 years between the eldest child, Tom, and myself. She had the thirteenth child four years later when she was 45. Three of the children died, and two of my brothers died in the last war. Violet died in infancy from one of the childhood diseases, and my twin brother died when he was about six months old, from diaorrhea. She wasn't able to breast-feed both of us and she got some milk from the welfare that didn't agree with him. I imagine it was a sort of enteritis. He most probably died of dehydration, I'd have thought. A sister called Lily died following chicken pox. She got a pneumonia and that was a tragedy. I remember the Saturday. We were all sent out to the park – we weren't to come back till a certain time and her word was rule, you did as she said – and when we came back Lily had died and my mother had laid her out on the front room table. We hadn't realised that she was so ill. I think she'd had a doctor, but there was no suggestion of her going to hospital. Women looked after their dying children at home. I remember my mother feeling so sad. Lily was eight. It was hard, whereas, I think when babies died there was nearly an acceptance of that – babies died, and that was part of life, you know...

We lived in a little two-up, two-down in Great Yarmouth, in Fox's Passage next door to a fish-curing place. They were little tiny terraced houses, all up the nooks and corners, and they all had big families living in those tiny houses. As the children got older, they had to move out 'cause there were only two bedrooms...

There were eight of us in a double bed, a brass bed, four at the top and four at the bottom. And before that, I can remember sleeping between my mother and father. I have vague memories of them, you know...they were making love. Yes, I couldn't have been very old. So the youngest ones obviously stayed in their bed.

I can remember my mother sitting at the table on Mondays, which was washing day...the big copper...she'd have been up at four o'clock getting this copper full of

boiling water and I was sent to get one pound of corned beef,
which was then extremely cheap. And we'd have it with
mashed potatoes and piccalilli. And that was Monday
morning. You sat at the table with all the sheets hanging
round you. You'd push the sheets away. All ten or twelve
of you sitting round the table. And sometimes we'd have
two rabbits from the market place for, say threepence, and
they'd go into a big oval pot on the coals – a great big
rabbit stew.

She was a good manager. She used to make clothes for
us all out of second-hand clothes – all the boys' trousers
made out of second-hand skirts and coats. She was always
knitting or sewing...

My dad was a fisherman but when the fishing all
collapsed in the Depression of the 1920s, they couldn't sell
the fish or the boats and the big companies came in... He
finished up a labourer by the time I was born. My father
was a very quiet, accepting sort of personality, which was
unusual amongst fishing folk, but my mother was a little
Geordie woman and she was a fighter, you see. She had this
big thing – she didn't want any of her children to have dead-
end jobs in the fishing or holiday season, or casual work –
she had a big thing that they'd all get decent jobs, not blind-
alley jobs. So they all went into apprenticeships. My mother
really wanted us all to get out of the situation there. She
put a lot of energy and ambition into it. She was a great
character.

As a little boy of four or five, I can remember her being
called out and it was either for laying people out or going
to a birth. They were the two main things. I do know my
mother never slept more than four or five hours all her
married life. That was mostly because she'd be called out.
They'd come and rattle on the window, you know, and
she'd put her head out the window and they'd say 'Will you
come?' And mum would go. There was people who couldn't
afford the midwife. The midwife, I think, was five shillings.
That, I think, was standard for delivery. People couldn't
afford five shillings so they'd come to my mother and
they'd give her whatever they could. This would be early
1930s that I remember, but she'd probably been doing it
for years. I think she got whatever they could afford to give
her. It might have been sixpence or a shilling. But she'd
always go. My memory is that babies always came at night-

time, but older children and next-door neighbours would look after me when she got called out.

She also went out to work, washing up and that in the cafes in the summer holiday season. Anything! She scrubbed steps, took in washing... And besides doing that, she used to cut people's hair for a ha'penny. And lay out dead bodies when people died, for sixpence. I think people came to her for advice. Apart from the house being all full of family, it was always full of other people coming. I suppose anyone who had any sort of hospital knowledge, I mean they were looked upon as having something to offer. You must remember people were very uneducated. My mother was educated. One good thing about her father dying was that when she was made a ward of court it was stipulated that the uncle had to send her to school. This was before the Education Act, so my mother had some education when most women didn't get any. She would have had a smatter of nursing from working in the fever hospital, and would have learned how to lay out bodies there. You were lucky if about a third of them survived in there, so she would have got plenty of experience. She may well have also learned things about nursing from my aunt, who was the village nurse.

She used to do painting and decorating too. They used whitewash then, or blue rinse – what we'd call emulsion paint now. The women did all the decorating – the men were out at sea, fishing. I can't ever remember my father doing anything in the house. He went out fishing and then he was in the pub. He had nothing to do with the children. We used to meet my father on a Sunday night on the prom! [promenade] Local people walked along the prom on Sunday nights in their best outfits – navy-blue serge suits, a white silk scarf and a cap – and we'd meet my father as though he was a stranger. We'd all be sitting on the prom seats, and he'd come up and give us a ha'penny each! Then off he'd go to the pub. Really, he was a total stranger to me. But that wasn't unusual... All the men spent all their free time in the pub.

Oh yes, she resented it. Continually. She nagged him from morn till night. But he needed it. I don't think he ill-treated her. In fact, I can't remember him losing his temper. I think he was too placid. I never saw him drunk. He gave her about half his wages and then the rest was for his tobacco and drink. My mother resented all that money going into beer that should have gone into the family. And we resented him, too, as we grew up. We had no respect for him. I can't say we were unhappy as children, but we were very hard up.

She didn't have a very happy relationship with the trained midwives. You can imagine how the midwives saw her. I mean, there was this unqualified person (in her eyes)... But when I came along there was some sort of Charity Midwife, and my mum knew her well because I remember meeting her in the market place and her asking about me and my younger sister. So obviously, you see what happened? I think they just sort of cooked their argument. They must have done. I think she must have stopped going out around the time when the Second World War came. By then, there were more trained nurses around, and so things began to change, and of course by then there was legislation...

I don't think she ever worked with doctors. No, you only called a doctor really if you were dying. I remember she had this varicose ulcer all her life, and if she went to the doctor she would have to pay, so she wouldn't go. Whereas my father had a penny thing on his pay, like an insurance to the local hospital. The men got that, but the wives never got anything! She had this great big ulcer, enormous great thing on her leg. I think she caught it on the fourth or fifth pregnancy on a bottom latch, you know, varicose veins and that... And she had that most of her life. I remember her going to a Chinese doctor who advised her to put it in a bucket of salt water. And that was the best thing that ever did anything ('cause she tried all sorts and that) but the interesting thing is when it nearly got healed she'd get thrombosis and phlebitis. As long as it was discharging, she was all right. I remember bandages and the smell of it from early on.

She died in the late 1950s, when she was about 73. My dad died two or three years later. Florrie and I were there when she died, and we both laid her out together. We were both nurses. The interesting thing was her skin was absolutely beautiful. She'd had all those pregnancies and that varicose ulcer for years, and yet she had a lovely skin. It was the last thing we did together. We sort of washed her. We did it as a last thing for her, really.

My mother was a real personality, this tiny little Geordie. She was a go-getter.

References

1. Little, Bob, *Go Seek Mrs. Dawson. She'll know what to do – The Demise of the Working-Class Nurse/Midwife in the Early Twentieth Century*, unpublished thesis, Sociology Dept., University of Essex, 1983.
2. Campbell, Janet, *Report on Public Health and Medical Subjects – The Training of Midwives*, HMSO, 1923, p.24.

3 Midwives in pre-NHS Britain

I'm glad I chose that profession. It's lovely. But you had to
be dedicated to it. It's very hard work.

Once midwifery was placed firmly in the hands of a professional
body, the Central Midwives Board (CMB), in the first decades of
this century, a strict supervisory and plenary apparatus ensured
that most working-class women were excluded from training
and practice. This chapter explores the working lives of the 'new'
certified midwives who worked in the 1920s, 1930s and 1940s.

Training

The training for midwives was lengthened progressively
throughout the first half of the century. By 1938, it lasted 24
months for unqualified women and twelve months for those
already trained as nurses. Although small grants or allowances had
been available from the Treasury for some student midwives
since 1919, they barely covered basic living expenses. In the
1920s, 1930s and 1940s, midwifery training was still an impossibility for most working-class women since student midwives still
had to pay for their own equipment, uniforms, examination fees
and, in some cases, for their tuition. However, sometimes an
agreement was reached with the hospital whereby these things
would be paid for by the student in a manner such as that
described by Nellie H., who did direct-entry midwifery training
(for non-nurses) in 1926:

> When I decided to do midwifery, I went to Plaistow
> Maternity Hospital. It was a very good training school and
> I really enjoyed it ever so much. Now I believe it's shut up
> – isn't that a shame? If we didn't pay to be a midwife, we
> had to stay on another six months and teach the little nurses
> that were on the district. That's what I did you see. You had
> to pay ten pounds – that was a lot for me – to get in. Once

you were in, you were OK. You got all your meals and everything was done for you, but we didn't get our uniform or our instruments or anything. We had to buy all those ourselves.

Mary W., who had already trained as a nurse, paid for her training by working without payment for six months *before* commencing the midwifery course in 1931. As she explains:

When I did my midwifery training I was going to be married and so I had to go to Bradford, which was the cheapest place. I went to this nursing home and gave my SRN [State Registered Nurse] experience to her in return for the midwifery training. No salary for six months. And at that time midwives were scarce. So how on earth they got away with not paying a salary... Mind you, in those days of course, nursing was a vocation. You were never encouraged to look upon it as a job, or a means of getting money.

Occasionally, working-class women would gain access to midwifery training by working in the fever hospitals where people with infectious diseases were isolated. This process was described by Ken W., a nurse whose mother was a handywoman and whose sister Florence managed to become a midwife against all the odds:

It's interesting that many of the midwives, particularly working-class midwives, got into it through the fever hospitals because it was made very difficult for them to train to be midwives. It was very expensive – they couldn't afford the uniform and books, and a lot of them couldn't afford the schooling to take the exams.

Whereas, with the danger of working in the fever hospitals and TB hospitals, they'd take anybody. It was a way in. And they got some nursing experience there.

My sister Florence had to leave school aged 14 as we all did. She was working as a maid in a boys' boarding school in Yarmouth in the late 1920s, but then she got caught up with the Salvation Army – by the evangelist thing – and was accepted at their training college in Camberwell. The headmaster and his wife at the boys' school were sympathetic to her wanting to train with the Salvation Army, so for a while she continued to receive the same pay from them, but an extra amount was put aside for her so that she could leave with an extra lump sum.

Florence won a scholarship. My mother couldn't afford
to let her go to the hospital. Couldn't afford the uniform
or the books. She was a bright girl. And that's how she got
into midwifery.

They never got paid as nurses in the Salvation Army
and however poor my mother was, she used to save up and
send Florence a postal order for a shilling.

Florence, herself, describes the strain imposed on working-
class women who found a way to enter midwifery training, an issue
that several other midwives commented on:

When I went off to start my training, I was very fearful. You
always felt as though you were inferior not having had the
education. Although you had other experience that those
nurses hadn't in life and that, you didn't have the head
knowledge.

Florence, like many midwives of the time, was driven by her
religious conviction, her sense of 'calling'. She once wrote to a
friend:

I never lose sight of my humble beginnings – I sometimes
wonder and feel it was presumption on my part to think
or expect that I could be used as a Salvation Army officer,
but it is equally wonderful to realise how God can, and does,
use and fit the most unlikely person, once that life has been
fully and unreservedly dedicated to His service.

All the midwives we interviewed referred to midwifery as a
vocation. Esther S. described how the Second World War gave her
the opportunity to fulfill her childhood ambitions:

I lived and worked in the same area of Portsmouth that I
was born in. I hadn't had a higher education. It was the war
that gave me the opportunity to do training. I got called
up. Ever since I used to play nurses with my dolls – bits of
rag as bandages, always making them better – I wanted to
train to be a nurse. My mother said that it was there, right
from those early days. But then, of course, there was no
opportunity. We were quite poor. We lived in a 'two-up and
a two-downer' so we had very little cash. My father was an
asthmatic so for every year there was three months he
never worked. They were the days where you didn't have
no back-up – if you didn't have any money, you didn't eat,
unless you had a good mother like I had that saved a bit

for the rainy day. So when I got to 14, I had to go out to work. There was no way that I could be educated. I say today, 'I do wish I'd had higher education, how wonderful it is!' You people don't know how lucky you are not being pushed out to work at 14.

I had no way of doing higher education. I left school and I went to work as an 'under children's nurse'. I worked with two nannies – a 'Princess Christian' and a 'Truby King' [different schools of thought and nursery nurse training] – quite different ideas. One believed in warmth and one would bathe the baby in front of an open window!

Now, when the war came, there was an opportunity to nurse even though you had no qualifications. You had to take a hospital exam – sort of general knowledge – that's how I got through. I volunteered. They were asking for people to go and nurse because of the war. There was this big notice in the hospital – a picture of a naval nurse with a big hat that gave the image of a nurse – and it said, 'WHY NOT JOIN US? – COME IN NOW', or something like that. It was a booking office. I said to my mother, who was taking me up there for treatment for my ears, 'Come on, let's go in and see what it's all about'. And I said to the man, 'I want to nurse'. I think he could tell how keen I was so he pointed me in the right direction. And that's how I got called up. I did the SEN training [State Enrolled Nurse training, a less academic course than the SRN, State Registered Nurse training course]. I loved it, loved it!

When they started up a midwifery school, Matron asked me if I'd like to do my training and I said, 'Oh yes'. I wanted to learn and I was so keen. I didn't want to go out when the other girls did, I just wanted to stay in, go over me notes and study. As soon as we came off duty, my friend – who was like me and from up North – and I, we'd say, 'Let's go and have a bath', and then one night we'd go to her room, one night we'd go to mine and we both went onto the bed and we'd study. There's quite a bit to learn isn't there? So that's what we did.

Other midwives described having to learn long chunks of textbooks by rote. This situation persisted throughout the 1950s, 1960s, and 1970s. There was little encouragement to question or debate issues. In effect, in pre-NHS days, as now, much of the learning took place while on placement in the community. The quality of the learning experience depended to some extent on the teaching skills of the community midwife and the relationship between student and teacher. Esther S. described the limitations imposed by class differences between her and her somewhat aloof community midwife:

> My midwife, Mrs T., she was very prim. She had a daughter named Deirdre – 'Deirdre', I thought, 'What a name!' She used to say it like 'Dayahdray'. [posh accent and laughter] And I'm so ordinary and there's this 'Deirdre' at boarding school and everything. Every morning we'd sort the work out, which meant that yours truly did the work and she'd come in and organise me. 'Oh, yes...yes, nurse...' [autocratic tone of voice] She had no sense of humour and she was very proper.

An authoritarian approach to midwifery teaching was described by many of the midwives we interviewed. These extracts from the unpublished autobiography *Storks Nest* by midwife Mary Thomson, vividly describe the first days of training at Rotten Row Hospital, Glasgow, in the early 1930s:

> And then rustling along the corridor she (the tutor) came. Like a starched and goffered advertisement for somebody's laundry, she swooped down upon us with perfection streaming from the crown of her small, white cap to the bows on her highly polished shoes. Her long, straight back was held stiff and unyielding, and she bristled all over with efficiency. It flew from her like electric sparks and shocked us into breathless wonder. She looked down her long, thin nose at us, and like the Ancient Mariner 'she held us with her glittering eye'. Her gaze wandered over each of us in turn, and what she saw didn't seem to please her much for she shook her head sadly and managed to sap the last ounce of self respect that had survived the onslaught of Sisters Lindsay and Martin... 'Well, now that you are here, I hope you are prepared for hard work and study', she said, as if she had finally made up her mind to make the best of a bad job. She spoke quickly and her words tumbled over each other like a cataract. 'I hope you all have your textbooks and copy books ready for your first class tomorrow morning at nine o'clock sharp and remember, I don't tolerate latecomers to lectures and tutorials, which will be arranged for your off-duty periods, and except for illness, no excuse will be taken for missing any one of them, and don't forget you are here to learn and I am here to teach

and if any of you are not prepared to comply with my methods you would be better to say so now and take yourselves off before it is too late, and now if you are all ready, I'll take you round the hospital'.

The next day she continued by proceeding 'to give us a short talk'. She began by criticising the way we had put on our uniforms and said we looked like a set of trollops. We would have to tighten up here and let down there, and as for our hair, that just about gave her a fit. We must all get it pinned tightly back from our faces and we were not to come into her lecture room looking like a set of street women.

Mary's high ideals of becoming a 'ministering angel on a mission of mercy' were soon shattered:

What did I find? I found what every other nurse finds in those first few weeks – that scrubbing, cleaning, polishing, sluicing, bed-panning, and who the hell do you think you are and what the devil are you doing here attitude from seniors, are the basic laws on which ministering angels are created... The new pupil is always beneath the notice of seniors and superiors. She is just a pair of hands for thrusting mops and dusters into and a pair of feet for scampering up innumerable flights of stairs and trekking miles and miles of corridors. She is Sister's sore head and Staff Nurse's pain-in-the-neck, and if she never had an inferiority complex before, she will certainly develop one before the first week is over.[1]

Midwifery training was clearly physically demanding and, it would appear, intellectually unstimulating. Midwives described a situation in which most formal teaching took place in off-duty periods. This could mean spending a day at lectures having had no sleep the previous night. Student midwives were left to work on their own from early on in their training, particularly on the district, and all the midwives said that this was a most valuable preparation for 'being a practitioner in your own right'.

Organisation of services

In the 1920s, once a midwife qualified, she could work in a variety of settings, including maternity hospitals (voluntary hospitals); in maternity departments of Poor Law Infirmaries (about to be renamed Local Authority or Municipal Hospitals under the Local Government Act of 1929); maternity departments of large Board of Governor hospitals, and in small maternity homes and newly built small hospitals. She could also work as a district midwife employed by local authorities; as a municipal midwife employed by nursing associations; as an independent (self-employed) practitioner; or, finally, attached to large teaching hospitals.[2]

The midwives we interviewed had worked in many of these areas. At the beginning of her midwifery career, Mary W. worked as an independent midwife on the district in the Yorkshire mining town where she grew up. As today, independent midwives would have to buy all their equipment, and the financial returns could be precarious since they were dependent on the number of bookings available. However, in the early 1930s, independent midwifery was the only option available to Mary W., as she explains:

> One of the reasons I went on to the district was because at that time no married woman, unless she was a widow, was employed in a hospital. [This was because midwives had to live in the nurses' home.] District midwifery was the only thing you could do – or district nursing. As a married midwife, it was the only thing left for me to do. But I never really wanted to go back into hospital once I got used to the district because there's a lot to be said for being an independent practitioner. Of course, the supervisor used to come round, but not very often, and you were your own boss in a way – got used to your own village, your own practice and doctors. We were on call 24 hours a day – if you got a call in the night, you still had to do your day's work the next day. In my biggest year, I did 99 cases, but usually about 80. It varied according to population. It was very satisfying being an independent practitioner...

In pre-NHS days, community midwives who were not working independently were employed by nursing associations, as retired midwifery tutor Mollie T. explains:

> Prior to '48, there were many charitable and religious organisations who contracted to the local authority to provide a midwifery service. In the 1930s we lived in a small village on the Kent coast, and we had there what was called a Jubilee nurse. These Jubilee nurses were women who

were selected from the villages, as being competent and sent to train at Plaistow Maternity Hospital as midwives. They were given a smattering of nurse training and sent back to their villages and the money that paid for this came out of Queen Victoria's Diamond Jubilee Fund. You know, their safety record was quite excellent.

In our village, she was always called either by her surname, or 'the Jubilee'. She had got terrible 'white leg' which must have been from childbirth followed by pelvic infection, and she used to get around the village on her own two feet, puffing and blowing and she must, at the time I remember, have had a heart condition, for she was always distinctly blue on exertion. And my mother always used to tell me to go and get a chair for Mrs So-and-so. Most people said, 'Oh, the Jubilee's here. Get a chair for her leg'.

She used to cover quite an area, at least two other villages along a seven-mile strip of the coast. She must have got there either by lifts or people coming to get her. She was in no state to cycle.

When Elsie B. worked as a district midwife in Devon in the 1930s, she was employed by a Nursing Association:

I'm only talking about Devon now, but other counties were the same. You had a Devon County Committee, which was based at Exeter. A county medical officer used to deal with the midwifery and you also had a midwifery inspector, and one for health visiting. You then had nursing superintendents – who you now call nursing officers and all sorts of funny names! We had a very good one and two assistants. But each area had its own local nursing committee. They used to collect subscriptions from people who belonged to this area. The people then got a free service for general nursing services. They paid, if I remember rightly, about one pound and five shillings for each confinement if they were members of the Nursing Association. And then we got our pay from the Association.

You were on full call with half a day a week off and three weeks holiday a year in those days. It used to work out about 90–100 deliveries a year. The most deliveries I did in one day was four in 24 hours. In all I delivered over 2,000 babies. You did the antenatal, delivery and full postnatal nursing, so you followed the women all through, which was nice. One area I worked you had 28 miles of road in the parish and you rode a bicycle.

With the coming of the Second World War, Nellie H. changed from private practice to becoming a 'council midwife':

> After I'd finished my training and worked for a while on the district, my sister asked me to come and join her working at Leigh-on-Sea in Essex. We had our own private business there, nursing and midwifery. We were there for quite a few years but then, of course, the war came. I didn't want to stay there doing nothing much in particular 'cause there wasn't much work, so I said to her, 'Well, I think I'm going to try to get a job somewhere. What about you Rosie?' 'Oh, I'm going to stop here and look after my mothers, never mind about the war', she said. I applied to the council. They were always glad to get hold of anyone those days. I s'pose we'd got the reputation because when the doctor from Southend-on-Sea came to see us, he said, 'Would you like to be evacuated with about 50 mothers?' So I said, 'Oooh – well, I don't know, I s'pose I could manage it'. 'Oh yes', he said, 'You've got a very good reputation here you know'.

These reminiscences give an indication of some of the advantages and disadvantages of midwifery practice before the establishment of the NHS. Midwives worked long hours with little time off, but in return they had the satisfaction of providing continuity of care for their clients using all their midwifery skills.

Payment for maternity services

Home births were cheaper than hospital births and, subsequently, they had lower status as far as some people were concerned. Middle-class women tended to opt for the maternity home or hospital care, presumably on the assumption that higher fees assured better care. Edie B. remembers the charges in the maternity home where she worked in the 1920s:

> It cost £2.10s in the maternity home, unless they went into a different section of the home which was slightly done up – a few more pictures on the walls, that sort of thing.

In Nellie H.'s private nursing home in the south of England just before the Second World War, the financial arrangements were as follows:

> We used to charge £5 every time a baby was born – £5 and the mothers stayed in a fortnight. We looked after them night and day – £5 – for everything! The middle-class women paid the same but they gave you good presents!

Private enterprise flourished in the private nursing home where Mary W. worked during her training in the early 1930s:

> This nursing home belonged to the matron herself, you know. She was the proprietor, and there we had various prices for rooms. And the women in the most expensive room never went home before a month. Matron used to stand at the bottom of the bed and she would say, 'You know the doctor and I have been having a little talk and he thinks you'd be much better if you stayed another fortnight'. More money, you see!

Women who could afford the fee often chose to book the services of a doctor for a home birth. In the early part of the century, problems arose when a doctor needed to be called in an emergency and people could not afford to pay the fee. After 1919, a system operated whereby the local authority was obliged to pay the doctor's fee in the first instance and would recover the costs later from the patient if possible. Before 1919, midwives were forced to pay the fee themselves when their clients could not afford it – or else face disciplinary proceedings and possible removal from the register if they did not fulfill the requirements of the rules by sending for medical aid. Elsie B., a district midwife working in Devon, recalls:

> A lot of these people didn't book a doctor. The farming people, or people in the money, they booked a doctor very often, but the ordinary workman couldn't afford one, so you sent a medical aid form if you wanted the doctor – but you didn't send unless you wanted him. If you sent a medical aid form, the county paid his fee. That's why the poorer people didn't book a doctor because they knew they could get him if they were in trouble. They relied on the midwife and the midwife had to have sense enough to know when a doctor was needed.

Working as a salaried midwife for a nursing association in the 1920s did not necessarily guarantee a living wage. Many letters to *Nursing Notes* (the midwives' professional journal) bear witness to that fact. The following is an extract from a letter written in November 1920, by a midwife on a salary of £84 a year:

> I was hoping to invest in a pair of new shoes as I have not had any since last year, and these are beginning to be leaky, but it is impossible. My cotton frocks I have had for three years, and these are so patched that I am afraid that they will fall to pieces in the wash. My rainproof coat is getting so thin that it will not be rainproof any longer. My district is a large one. I have three villages and the nearest doctor is four and a half miles away, and the road is a very bad, uphill one to get to him. There is no telephone in either village and only one telegraph office which opens at 9 a.m. and closes at 7 p.m. The roads in the winter are awful; sometimes one cannot use the bicycle as there is too much mud...
>
> It is lonely as she [the midwife] cannot join in anything socially, as there is always something to pay... I cannot afford to join the Women's Institute or anything else, and it is hard to see everybody else go off to the local enter- tainment and have to stay behind because of the expense.
>
> It is not pleasant by any means to be called up at all hours in the night and go through woods and fields to cases – in all weathers. I should not advise any woman to take up midwifery, especially in a rural district, unless she had private means, as she would be almost a hermit because she could not afford to join in any social pleasures, and she would always be shabby and in debt. No, life is not sweet to a rural midwife, with the spectre of want always before her eyes.
>
> There is one thing that I should like to tell you about, and that is the snobbery of the richer people in the country villages towards the village nurse. I think that is another reason why a midwife should not settle for very long in the country. Perhaps it is because the salary is so small that the big subscribers can afford to treat her so. They think they are helping her out of charity. [These are the people who would sit on the panel of the nursing association employing the midwife.][3]

The development of a salaried profession

The Midwives Act of 1936 brought about fundamental changes to the organisation of maternity services. For some time, the midwife had been seen as the key link between childbearing women and the ever-increasing system of state-funded benefits, introduced in response to appalling infant and maternal mortality statistics (*see* Chapters 1 and 2). The state needed to create a new system that would bring the majority of midwives – who were working as private practitioners – under the tighter control of local authority co-ordination so that they could be their agents.

Under the 1936 Midwives Act, local councils were charged with providing an adequate, salaried domiciliary midwifery service, either directly or through voluntary organisations. This meant that, apart from those midwives who chose to work independently, all practising midwives would be salaried with guaranteed 'off duty' and annual leave. Although the clients would no longer have to pay the midwife directly, unless there was great hardship, they would have to pay the local authority for midwifery care. The new system was a great relief to midwives such as Mary W., who had been struggling to make a living as an independent practitioner:

> Of course, before 1936, your income was very precarious because you had what you earned. The amount of deliveries you got was the amount of money you got. I was charging 30 shillings. I've always been paid, but sometimes by instalments, because people hadn't a lot of money in the early 1930s. A lot of the men were only working half a week, then half a week on the dole, so they had very little income and there was a lot of poverty.
>
> The 1936 Act said that the local authorities had to provide midwives for the people in its area. Well, the posts were advertised and we all applied. In fact, it helped the local authority to weed out the ones they didn't want. It gave them more control over us. Some midwives didn't get jobs and it caused a lot of hard feeling. There were four of us who had been practising independently in this area and I was one of the two who were chosen. One of the ones not chosen was a newly qualified SCM [State Certified Midwife] – she was a direct entrant [non-nurse] – and the other one had her SRN [State Registered Nurse] qualification but she hadn't endeared herself to the authorities. She got a job the

following year, but she never forgave me in all the time we worked together for getting the first job! She was a real thorn in my side. The re-organisation caused a lot of friction. Some of the ones that didn't get jobs took compensation – there was a scheme for that – but they didn't get much at all.

After the 1936 Midwives Act and until the NHS was set up in 1948, midwives working for a nursing association or local authority were still responsible for collecting their fees, a task they described as extremely difficult when people could not afford to pay. In fact, many midwives said that the best thing about the advent of the NHS was that they no longer had to collect payment from their clients. Katharine L. explains the financial arrangements that existed in the late 1930s in East Anglia:

> In an area like this, patients would pay into three funds. There was one where you paid 1d or 2d a week to the hospital, so that if you went into the hospital you didn't have to pay. There was another one for the District Nursing Association. That was 2d a week. And then there was the HSA [Hospital Saving Association, a health insurance scheme]. And so if we had a patient that was paying 2d a week into the District Nurses Association and she was going to have a baby, instead of having to pay us £2.10s for her delivery and aftercare, she only had to pay thirty bob [30 shillings]. They didn't pay us; they paid the Association. But of course we had to collect it from the patient for the Association and that was hard.

Midwives and doctors

In pre-NHS days, midwives often found themselves competing with doctors for maternity cases. Rivalry between midwives and the medical profession had existed for centuries, and is well documented in Jean Donnison's *Midwives and Medical Men*.[4] Early midwifery campaigners such as Alice Gregory steered midwifery along a course that publicly acclaimed the superiority of the medical profession:

> If we are unduly aggressive in our dealings with doctors, who are not very enthusiastic about our arrival on the scene to start with, we help to put the clock back and discredit our profession. Of course, there are some irreconcilables among the medical profession, with whom one

can do nothing. I grieve to say I have heard of one lately, whose determined opposition has caused the abandonment of the midwife's work in a country village; but I think that such implacable hostility is the exception if the midwife treats them respectfully as her professional superiors.[5]

Arguably, the subordination of the profession was reinforced by legislation that ensured that the services of a doctor had to be employed in all situations where there were complications – a ruling that also ensured a regular income for the medical profession. The parallels between the subordination of the all-female midwifery profession and the position of women in society are obvious. In spite of social pressures, most midwives we interviewed saw themselves as equals to doctors. Many, such as Edie B., who worked alongside male doctors in a maternity home, described positive working relationships:

> On the whole, we got on well with the doctors. Mind you, you didn't let them get away with things. I remember one woman, she'd been in labour quite a long time and the doctor came to see her and he said, 'You must pull yourself together. It's *your* baby. *You're* having it, and *you* must do the work'. You know the sort of attitude. And the woman said, 'Can I have a cup of tea?' Doctor said, 'Not until you've had your baby'. So I said, 'Well, anyone who's doing such hard work deserves a nice cup of tea'. She got her cup of tea!
>
> I once did a forceps because the doctor collapsed! Well, it wasn't good for her to do it. She was on the point of collapse. 'Oh, I don't feel very well. Do you think you could manage?' I said, 'Well, if you tell me the position and where exactly to put the instruments, where to feel, I'll have a go, but you must take responsibility'. However, the baby was all right. I was so relieved. I went about with an imaginary medal on my chest! I enjoyed that, the feeling of power, you know. No, our doctors were very nice. They respected us and treated us like equals. They trusted us and you thanked that feeling of trust.

Elizabeth C. also recounted tales of putting on forceps, in her case because of the lack of experience of many of the doctors who arrived when she sent for help at home births:

You often put the forceps on for them because a lot of the doctors didn't know what they were doing. They didn't sort of know which end was which! They hadn't done it, you see, so they depended on you. They may have been there, responsible for whatever cropped up, but that didn't always ease your mind because something could be done that shouldn't be done.

District midwife Margaret A. remembered the outrage and frustration she felt over one doctor's practice:

This was the most terrible doctor. She was booked by this girl having her first baby and it was coming a bit before its time. She had a fairly long labour and the doctor arrived, did an examination, put forceps on and dragged out a little four-pound baby. She tore the girl's cervix and killed the baby. There was a lot of talk about this afterwards and Kath heard that the doctor had been telling people that it was my fault – 'the midwife didn't send for her soon enough'. With her next baby, she booked the same doctor. It was a normal birth at term this time, but she had a retained placenta. After an hour, we had to call this doctor out. She came in and inverted her uterus! [Pulled the uterus out through the vagina.] The poor soul was taken up to the general hospital where they managed to peel the placenta off the uterus – though it was firmly adherent – but the girl died of shock. It was an avoidable death. But that doctor was a terrible liar and she always tried to put the blame on anyone else.

Midwives engaged by wealthy families to live in often found themselves playing a servile role to the doctor whose services were also engaged. Midwife Elsie K. remembers:

There was one case, she was a doctor's wife and although I'd been hired to live in, she was to be delivered by another doctor, a specialist. In those days, we often had a coal fire in the bedroom and I used to put the rubber gloves the doctors gave me to boil up, in a little pan on the fire. On this occasion, it was a second baby and I knew it was nearly ready to deliver, so I let his gloves boil for a couple of minutes and then I handed them back to him. And he said, 'I like my gloves boiled for ten minutes, Nurse'. So I said to myself, 'All right Sir, you shall deliver this baby without gloves'. And I put them back on the fire. And of course, he had to deliver without gloves because the baby was imminent. You see, *I'd* been watching the patient!

By the time the NHS was set up nearly half a century after the first Midwives Act, a strong precedent had been established in Britain. Midwives were the recognised practitioners of normal childbirth, and doctors were only called to labours with complications. By 1948, the power struggle between professionals had shifted away from the birthing room and into the antenatal clinic. Mary W. saw this period as a turning point in midwifery:

> The midwife's status has gone down such a lot recently. It started around the time of the NHS Act, I think, when the doctors started doing more and more antenatal care and the midwives said, 'Oh well, the doctor gets paid for it – he'll do it'. Instead of sticking up for their own status, they let their status go, and that's where the midwives started to go down.

Day-to-day work

The midwives we interviewed all had vivid memories of their day-to-day working lives. Although the work was demanding and not easy to organise in the days before cars, telephones and radio-pagers, they all described it with affection, humour and often a good deal of passion. For instance, Edie B., who worked mostly in nursing homes and hospitals, stated:

> It was a happy time. I'm glad I chose that profession. It's lovely. But you have to be dedicated to it. It's very hard work. Talking to you brings it all back. It was lovely.

District midwives' usual form of transport was either by bicycle or foot until well into the 1950s. Mary W. remembers these arrangements very positively:

> You missed a lot when you came off the bike. Although it was hard work you knew all the people along the way. All the shopkeepers knew you – 'There's the Nurse going along'. On your old bike, trundling along. Patients would be outside houses sometimes and shout, 'How are you? Got time to come in and have a cup of tea on your way back?' And things like that. You've lost a lot in the car.

On the other hand, sisters Katherine L. and Margaret A., who worked together on the district in East Anglia, found that bicycling became too arduous:

> We were on bicycles and then we had that terrible winter of '47 and we thought we can't go through another winter like this, so we went and told our committee – 'Sorry Dr. Allen I think we'll have to leave, we can't go through another winter like this'. And then we discovered that through one of our old patients, a General, we'd inherited £200. He'd given them £200 to buy the nurses a car – and they hadn't done a darn thing about it! However – we got a car. And we always had a car after that. We had a lot of clobber to carry around you know, bags, gas and air, oxygen, blocks to raise the beds up to save your poor old back [this would apply mainly to their practice after 1948].

Midwives were called to a birth by a knock on their door, usually from the husband or one of the children. In the day-time, when they were out doing their 'nursings' (postnatal visits), they would leave information as to their whereabouts. Margaret A. and Katherine L. recall:

> Every morning we would go out and write on a slate that was outside the front door. We would start with the first call and list them down to the bottom. If the labour happened during the day they would come round to the house, see the slate, take note, and come round and get us or find us. The slate was in a big sort of plastic bag so that if it rained the chalk didn't all get washed off. It worked well. But funnily enough, we found that most people start off labour at night.

Mary T. describes how people would come to the home she shared with midwife Elsie Walkerdine in order to call Elsie out to labours:

> In those days, Elsie kept the maternity box at home. One man came for Elsie – 'All right father', she said (for Elsie always called the patients 'mother' or 'father', never by Christian names). 'Take this and I'll be along in a minute'. I went with Elsie, and it was snowing. Up the High Street we walked and there was two people on the pavement as we were approaching. It was a policeman and this young man. 'Ah', he said. 'I'm glad you've come along, nurse. Tell

this copper what I've got in this parcel, will you? I don't bloody well know'. So the policeman turned round and said, 'Why didn't you tell me you'd been to get the midwife?' He said, 'You didn't ask! You asked me what I had in the box!'

Elizabeth C. remembers a messenger coming to the house she shared with her friend, another midwife. The labouring woman obviously had experience and knew that she was about to push the baby out (a phase of labour that midwives refer to as 'fully dilated'):

> The woman used to clean for my friend and I took this message from her. She said, 'She said to say she's fully DELIGHTED!' I knew what she meant and we had to hurry!

Fathers and children at births

Beyond calling out the midwife, it seems that fathers played virtually no role in the labour. On the whole, neither they nor the other children were present at the birth. Elizabeth C., who worked on the district in Battersea, explains:

> It was very rare for the fathers to be there, but they came in and out with anything you wanted. The men didn't want to be there and the wives didn't want them there either. But the women nearly always had their mums or a neighbour to help. Battersea was an area where they all helped one another. It was a tight-knit community.
>
> One lassie and her neighbour had fallen out over something or other and they hadn't spoken for ages. The day Mrs. B. went into labour, the neighbour come in and said, 'I'll take your Marion and look after her while you're in bed – but I haven't finished with you yet!' [laughs]

Mary T. used to accompany her friend, Elsie Walkerdine, to births in Deptford. Occasionally, Elsie would ask her to come and 'hold the girl's hand and encourage her', but on the whole she used to look after the husbands:

> Normally, I used to sit downstairs and keep the husband company, you know, chatting away – you usually found something to talk about. And all of a sudden you'd hear a little squeal and a bit later Elsie would appear and say, 'Father, you've got a nice baby boy!' I remember one bloke,

in the excitement he goes, 'I've got a boy, I've got a son!'
and he hit me on the back so hard he nearly knocked me
choppers out!

Josephine M. expressed strong feelings about the idea of men
being involved in childbirth:

> Oh, no, no, no! The husbands were never there when the
> babies were being born. I remember the fight I had with one
> dirty old devil. She, poor soul, had a baby every year and
> this was number nine or ten. He spent all their money in
> the pub, and was always in trouble with the cops. That was
> one of those cases where you couldn't take the maternity
> pack – you know the pack with all the pads and everything
> in it for the delivery – to the home in advance because he'd
> take it straight down to the pawn shop! This creature,
> what he used to do was pull the cloth across to see what
> was going on when she was having the baby – the dirty old
> dog! But it was sad, terribly sad. Oh no, you didn't want
> them there.

During labour, children would be banished from the house onto
the streets, or into the care of a neighbour or relative. Elsie B.
remembered a situation in the 1930s where no such support was
forthcoming:

> In a country district, there was a big house and the lady of
> the house was throwing a big party. Well, the poor butler's
> wife went into labour on the night of this big party and the
> lady of the house wouldn't release him or any of the other
> staff to help. She wasn't very thoughtful to the woman
> having a baby even though she was pregnant herself. So
> there was no-one to look after the woman's little toddler.
> But anyway, we managed. We had the toddler in the room
> all the time and she was perfectly all right. She was funny,
> really funny. Now I hear they let the children in...

Elsie K. bore the brunt of 'sibling displacement' when she was
hired to live in with a family in order to attend the mother – a
common practice in the 1920s and 1930s in middle-class circles,
particularly in rural areas:

> I didn't enjoy my first case at all. It was a third baby, and
> of course, I always had to be living in the house at the end
> of the pregnancy, waiting for the labour. I had to share a
> bedroom with this two-year-old and he used to wake early

and throw his toys at me to wake me up. He was very upset with life. I used to take him out in the afternoons to give the maid a break, and eventually it got better. But I didn't enjoy the experience because the husband was drinking himself to death, unfortunately. It wasn't a happy household.

Working hours

Mary T. remembers the restriction to Elsie Walkerdine's social life caused by the need to be accessible at all times:

If she went to the pictures, the little Picture Palace up the High Street (Deptford), they'd always know where she was sitting, so they could call her. She didn't have any off-duty, not like they do now. She was always on call, but in August – she never booked any confinements for August. That was her time off and then she'd take her aunt and uncle away. She went to Clacton religiously.

In pre-NHS days, 'off-duty' time was practically non-existent. Mary W. recalls:

I didn't get any time off at all when I was working on my own [as an independent midwife], of course, but then after I was employed by the council I got half a day a week off. I had one Christmas day off in all the time I was working, from when I started my training. You had very little time off. If you'd had a lot of deliveries – a lot of nights up, no-one made it up for you, you just had to go on and get it over and get your sleep when you could. I remember one week when I didn't see my husband to speak to. At the end of the week, he said, 'Oh, you still live here then, do you?' Yes, they come all together, babies, don't they, and they come in bad weather. When I was walking, if I had a booking at the far end of the district and it was snowing, a baby'd be sure to come.

Lack of 'time off' led to midwives working incredibly long hours, as Esther S. recalls:

One weekend I had seven babies single-handed and that's when I had that big baby (twelve and a half pounds!). That was the only time I've been so desperate. I was 'drunk' – I never understood the saying 'drunk with tiredness'

until then. I was high as a kite! I never went to my bed for
four nights and four days. I was fed in the houses with bits
of toast but I never went for my meals at all. From one to
another – sterilizing bowls in the houses as I went around.
And when I got home on the last day, my legs were so
swollen I could not put them on the bed. When I went in,
my mother said, 'At last, you're home. Where have you
been?' It was about 7 a.m. She heard me come in. I said, 'Oh
Mum, I don't think I can get up the stairs'. So she came
down and she pushed me up and said 'I'll go down and
make a cup of tea'. (I'll always remember this story.) And
when she came up I was laying on the floor. She said,
'You'll have to get on the bed 'cause you're going to sleep!'
I said, 'No, I'm too tired'. She said, 'Let me get some clothes
off for you'. She got me undressed, pushed me on to the
bed and I never woke up for 48 hours. I never passed urine,
I never woke for food, I never did anything, and my mother
was so frightened that she rang in the supervisor and said,
'She's just in a coma'. Supervisor said, 'Well, she's been
having lots of deliveries and everything. Go over and get
her midwife friend, get her down and see what she thinks'.
So she (my midwife friend) said, 'No, she's not in a coma,
she's just in a dead sleep'. And I never opened my eyes for
48 hours. And when I woke, I didn't know what time it was,
what day it was...

Besides the official demands of their work, midwives often did
a lot that was over and above the call of duty. Mary T., for
example, remembers her friend's dedication to midwifery:

Elsie's work was her life. It was 'her babies', and if somebody
paid her so much money a week, which they used to, and
they hadn't paid enough by the time the baby came, Elsie
couldn't turn round and say, 'Well, I'm sorry I can't come'.
That wasn't Elsie. Elsie used to turn round and make
allowance for it. And she was always knitting for the babies.
Some people would pay her in kind, like food and stuff,
especially when the war was on. Now, I do know that Elsie
exchanged her margarine for their butter because they
couldn't afford butter, people with children. The women
loved her. Really and truly she was idolized. The description of them people was 'she's an angel'.

One of Elsie's clients, Sissy S., remembers the care she received
from her:

I used to go round to see Nurse Walkerdine about once a month during my pregnancies...just to pay her half-a-crown off of me bill, which was £2 in all. No, she didn't listen to the baby's heart or nothing. She used to say, 'Well, how are you? Felt any movements yet?' – questions like that. And if you wasn't too good – 'Well, I'll be round and have a look at you'. That was all. Yes, if you wasn't well she'd take your blood pressure and that. She was right medical, and she knew every mortal thing what to look for. But I never had any trouble, thank God. They never examined you unless you weren't well. The only reason I went to see her was to pay off the bill. You could go and see her if you were worried about anything. There was no 'Wait a moment' with Nurse Walkerdine. If you went there, you saw her. Even if you went there when that nurse was having her dinner – 'Oh, I'm sorry Nurse Walkerdine, I didn't know you was having your lunch' – 'Well, come along in, it won't take a minute'. You wasn't put at unease, you know, that you'd disturbed her. She was a wonderful woman.

Midwives and mothers

Some of the midwives we interviewed were unusual in that, like Esther S., they were working-class women who practised in their own communities:

I lived and worked in the same area I was born in, went to school in. Therefore I watched the people, my friends, grow up. When they got married, I went to their weddings and then, of course, when they got pregnant I happened to have become the district midwife, so I was the midwife. And that to me was something super, really. Because I don't suppose in this day and age there's many people that live and work in their same area. That was really special. Excepting for the fact that although I was a friend I had to be their midwife, which was understood.

Wherever the midwives practised, they were anxious to include the element of professionalism that their training had taught them. Mary W. explains:

When I first started, an old doctor said, 'I'll give you a tip, nurse. Familiarity breeds contempt'. He had a marvellous bedside manner and he was greatly respected. And he said, 'Always keep your professional distance'.

Now I would never let them – even the people who had been to school with me and that sort of thing – never called me by my Christian name. I always sort of had my status and kept it. And they respected it. It was a good thing.

But I think they did look on me as a friend. I still see people and they like to see me. Nobody ever calls me 'Mrs W.' It's always 'Nurse W.' wherever I go. And even now that I've retired, they say, 'Eeegh! but I called you Nurse W.' And I say, 'Well, nobody ever calls me anything else'. They all knew me by that.

Most of the midwives we met spoke warmly of the women they had cared for, and of the relationships they had developed with them. Some were still in touch with 'their' mothers and babies, and indeed two of them were actually living in the home of a grown-up 'baby'. Elizabeth C. is one of those midwives:

I don't think they thought of me as just a midwife, more as a friend. Most of the kids and all, they used to call me 'Aunty Betty' – they still write to me as 'Auntie Betty', even the adults... I think there's a lot in being a personal friend to the person having the baby. You want a bit of sympathy and someone you can talk to just then. Not someone telling you, 'Now shut up. Stop making a noise'. I used to say, 'Shout if you want to dear, I won't take any notice'.

Mary W. delivered two generations in her Yorkshire village:

Yes, you had a lot of knowledge about the families and it was rather nice to go back and deliver the girls you'd already delivered. Sometimes I'd delivered both the father and the mother of the child that I was delivering then. It was nice to get to the second generation. And I almost got to the third generation. There was one girl and I'd delivered her and then her daughter, and then her daughter had a baby but she went into hospital for it because she was only young, but I did a lot of second generations.

As some midwives reminisce about the particular quirks of individual mothers, their attitudes might appear somewhat patronising, but a genuine affection came across during the interviews:

One mother in particular – she ended up with 13 [babies]. Now she started off, well, when we first came here she'd got four, three of her husband's and one, well, it could be anybody's. Then she started with a Greek. She left her husband and went and lived with a Greek, and she had three of his – we had 'em all didn't we, Kath. She had three Greeks. Then he went off to London and she took in a lodger. He was a man who left his wife and seven children, and he gave her five. She had them all at home. She wouldn't go into hospital. But we got very fond of her. She used to sit on the couch. I'd say, 'Now look, you go into hospital for this one, I'm not having you at home'. And she'd cry! (*Margaret A.*)

While Esther S. reported that she had never arrived too late for a delivery, Josephine M. who worked on the district in Croydon, implied that some women leave it too late to call the midwife on purpose. During our interview with her, it was sometimes hard to keep up with her rapid and expressive accounts of working life in the 1930s and 1940s, let alone derive historical information from her underlying insinuations:

Of course, some of them would send for the midwife when the baby was in the bed! And of course they'd tell you all sorts of nonsense – and you knew perfectly well that she wanted to have it in the bed because she didn't want to have us there.

You want to know why? Well now, say you're having a baby, do you want to have a lot of nurses fussing around you? Now do you? No, of course you don't. And anyway, there's midwives and midwives, isn't there? Well, there you are... And nothing ever happens. And there's lot of babies been born into the bucket, or in the toilet – and pick them up out of the toilet, and they're all right, aren't they? The cord may have snapped, but it doesn't always, and when a cord snaps it never bleeds. If a baby does fall, if it's a long cord, it won't snap. If it's a short cord, it might. But it's all right and the nipper's in the toilet and that's all there is to it! It's nothing, nothing. If it's a bit cold, wrap it up, feed it, Bob's your uncle, put it down the bottom of the bed. The mothers would keep them warm in the beds.

As Josephine M. said, 'There's midwives and midwives...' In fact, the testimony of most of the midwives we interviewed gave an impression of the very special relationships that can exist between women and their midwives. Many of them positively 'lit up' with pleasure as they relived their working lives. Elizabeth C. recalls:

> It was a vocation for me. I was in my element. People say, 'Oh, you can't have done', when I say I enjoyed every minute of it, even the up-at-nights, but it's true. You were doing something, you see. Once the fun began, you didn't feel tired, but you might come in in the morning and just fall into bed. But you'd find energy you didn't know you had.

Several midwives also remembered how intuition had played an important part in their work. Elizabeth C. strongly believes in the power of intuition:

> I do, yes. Oh, I do very much. I had a fair quantity of that. I always knew. I always knew when I was wanted straight away, you see. I can remember getting out of bed one morning for the telephone. I didn't know her. This wasn't my patient. It was somebody elses. And I said to my friend, 'I bet that baby's being born now'. And I got on me bike with me pants half on and I went down to this house off York Road, a long way from us, and lo and behold, the baby was coming all right and in a big hurry! My friend used to say that if I said something was happening she never dallied on it. In one case, she'd been in and out and there was nothing much doing. It was the next street to us and they sent up again for her. I said, 'I would go Anne, I would go, I wouldn't wait'. Anne left her breakfast there and off she went, just in time to catch the baby. I don't know what it is, just something or other that tells you what to do.

Midwives' personal lives

Most midwives we interviewed had been a midwife or nurse all of their working lives. They gave the impression that midwifery had been a dominating feature of everything they did. This was especially true for those who had remained single, some of whom had lived in the nurses' home until retirement. One midwife expressed her sorrow at being childless:

> I often wish I'd had a baby... Yes...but there it was...I chose the profession...

Midwife Mollie T. told us of situations in which unmarried midwives 'took home unwanted or orphaned babies' and brought them up as their own. Whether a formal adoption took place was not clear. (Adoption did not have legal status until 1926.) The prevalence of this practice was not made clear, either, but Mabel P., who worked as a midwife before training as a doctor in the 1910s, recalls combining professional and family life:

> I realised early that you couldn't work and do the things you wanted to do if you had a husband because that left you having babies – it was different then. Years later, I adopted (as babies) twin girls and a boy who was unrelated to the girls – and my family looked after them. My sister was housekeeper. So I managed to have children without having a husband and giving up my career.

Some midwives appeared to be clinging to memories of what they referred to as 'my babies'. One had been hired by wealthy families to 'live in' before and after the birth. She kept books full of memorabilia associated with these experiences. She appeared to be as proud of 'my babies' as if she had given birth to them herself.

Often we would be treated to lengthy accounts of what the babies wore, and sometimes we were given the impression that the babies were more important to the midwives than the mothers were. Indeed, there were a couple of midwives who were most disparaging about the mothers' ability to look after their children properly. They expressed pity for 'the poor wee mites' and there was an unspoken implication that they would have done better:

> Some of them were very careless, didn't care what their children did. I remember one baby being born on the floor in the ward, and of course its mother didn't even have the sense to get on the bed – just dropped it!

Mary T. reflected on the choices made by her friend, Elsie Walkerdine, with whom she lived for almost 40 years until Elsie died:

> Elsie loved the babies. Her babies were her life. I mean, early on, there was a local young man who sort of wanted to court her – you know how it was those days. But *no* – her work came first. He said, 'It sounds as though you'd prefer your work to me…' She said, 'I still want to bring babies into the world'. So she kept on her own all through life. She was never unhappy though because her work was her life.

Elsie's mother died soon after she was born and she was brought up by her uncle and aunt. They had no children and they doted on her – she was tied to their apron strings. They helped to pay for her to do midwifery – you didn't get it like you do today. On Boxing Day, 1940, I was living next door with my sister and I was invited in for a game of cards. I stayed the night 'cause there was no-one in at home, and I never went back to live with my sister. That was the start of a wonderful friendship. I never went anywhere without Elsie. I looked on her as like my mum.

Some midwives formed close relationships with other midwives, with whom they lived and shared their working and domestic lives over many decades. One of the authors grew up in a village where two women lived together as a much-loved and respected 'couple'. Together they covered all the district nursing, midwifery and health visiting in the area. In an era when midwives were expected to be totally dedicated to their vocation, such couples were seen as pillars of society who sacrificed marriage and children for the sake of their calling. Living together was, and is, seen as an ideal practical arrangement. The depth and personal importance of such relationships was also valued. It is not unusual to read acknowledgements of them in the obituary section of the *Midwives Chronicle*: 'Our sympathies extend to her lifelong companion and friend...'

In comparing the testimonies of midwives and mothers, it became obvious that although we had a strong impression of the midwives as workers, we had little sense of their personal lives. Esther S. was a notable exception and shared intimate experiences, such as the birth of her stillborn baby (*see* Chapter 11). In contrast to the midwives, mothers talked vividly about their feelings and personal experiences. This may reflect the fact that midwives often had to suppress their feelings in order to function as over-worked practitioners who needed to live up to an accepted image of professionalism.

The next few chapters explore in detail various aspects of child-bearing on women's lives and their effects on midwifery practice.

References

1. Thomson, Mary, *Storks Nest*, unpublished autobiography. We would like to thank Mary Thomson's son for allowing us to publish quotations from her book.

2. Towler, Jean and Bramall, Joan, *Midwives in History and Society*, Croom Helm, London, 1986, p.214.
3. *Nursing Notes*, November 1920, p.118.
4. Donnison, Jean, *Midwives and Medical Men*, Schocken Books, New York, 1977.
5. Gregory, Alice (ed.), *The Midwife: Her Book*, Frowde & Hodder & Stoughton, London, 1923, p.11.

4 Women's knowledge about 'the facts of life'

> Well, we were all green. I was as green as that bloody chair when I got married...

Talking with older women about their sex lives triggered many memories. Feelings of sadness and resentment about lack of knowledge were often expressed with a mixture of bitterness and a lively sense of humour. Women described situations where they knew very little about sex or how their bodies worked. They felt that this was typical of women who grew up in the first half of this century, regardless of class background or general education.

In those days, in fact up until the 1960s, there was, in effect, little or no sex education in schools and no open discussion of sexual matters in magazines or other media. Any allusions to sex in popular women's literature were heavily veiled in euphemisms. In *Agony Columns*,[1] Terry Jordan points out that it was not until the 1930s that there was any mention of sex and even then the advice was safely wrapped in obscure language. She quotes the 'agony aunt' writing in *Woman's Life*, 5 April 1930:

> In confidence.
>
> Dear Readers and Friends,
>
> There is no more difficult problem for a girl to settle, in her friendships with men, than this one, about which so many write to me. How much love-making should a girl permit? For I do feel very strongly that it is always up to the girl to set the standard. Nearly all men, even the nicest ones, will become too venturesome if they are allowed. It's just masculine nature – man is the hunter and must always take the lead. It is not a bit of good blaming them for it. A girl should concentrate rather on making any real liberties impossible.

STAND FIRM!

For she can. The matter is always in her hands, if she will only realise it and be firm. And the best way of being firm is never to allow the first little step, which seems so harmless and easy.

Of course, I am not suggesting that a girl should be a prude. When a man loves a maid it is natural that they should want to kiss and be alone together quite often. There are little ways of making love of which no sensible person disapproves – and there are other little ways which no girl who values her self-respect and her chances of marriage will ever allow.

I need not specify what these undesirable ways are. Every girl who is genuinely anxious to do the right thing and to come to her husband perfectly fresh and pure will recognise them, even if she has never met them before. However the man may coax or justify them, a little warning voice within her will cry 'Beware!'

MORE WILL BE ASKED.

The thing itself may seem quite pleasant and harmless. Taken alone, it is often both these things. But do realise that the man, whatever he may say or believe, won't be willing to stop there. One point gained, and in a week he is pleading for another. Always the hunter desires a further conquest. Readers often write and ask me, 'What does such and such form of love-making mean?' My dears, whatever it is beyond kissing, it means only one thing. It is just a step nearer the end nature had in mind when she made men and women. And that is why all such endearments should be kept until after marriage.

If a man cannot wait until then, he is not likely to make the girl happy after the wedding. There is another point. The girl who finds herself growing miserable and quarrelsome with her boy – or he with her – is often really the victim of this better-avoided kind of love-making. During the courtship stage, it excites without satisfying and is responsible for many a nervous breakdown and many a broken engagement.

So heed that little 'Beware!' when it rings in your mind.

Your sincere friend
Margaret[2]

More than three decades later in the 1960s, the advice and ethics expressed by this agony aunt were still forming the basis of the sex education received by the authors of this book. However, in the 1930s, the possibility of sex education for children was just beginning to be mooted in certain quarters. For instance, in *The Modern Woman's Home Doctor*,[3] a handbook that may have found its way into some of the better-off homes of the 1930s, there is a chapter entitled, 'What to Teach the Children about Sex'. However, it focuses on plants, insects and mammals, with only a short and unexplicit section on 'How You Began' that would certainly have left most children none the wiser.

Advice about sex had been available – albeit for a privileged minority – since 1918 when Marie Stopes first published *Married Love*.[4] Originally a doctor of botany, Marie Stopes was motivated by five years of unconsummated marriage to study every book on sex in the British Museum – involving texts in English, French and German. As a result of her research, Marie Stopes wrote a book that contained frank discussions of foreplay, clitoral stimulation and female orgasm. Stopes advocated an approach to sexual intercourse that took into consideration a woman's sexual response.

> The supreme law for husbands is: remember that each act of union must be tenderly wooed for and that no union should ever take place unless the woman also desires it and is made physically ready for it.[5]

Married Love was a best-seller but it certainly was not in general circulation and very few women would have had access to it. Even if they had managed to get hold of a copy, they may well have found its flowery language incompatible with the everyday reality of their lives:

> Welling up in her are the wonderful tides, scented and enriched by the myriad experience of the human race from its ancient days of leisure and flower-wreathed love-making.[6]

It was not simply lack of information that affected women. Mis-information was often employed, perhaps in an attempt to protect young people from reality. Sex was a taboo subject, so parents were doubly hampered in explaining the facts – not only by their own lack of knowledge and vocabulary but also by a deeply conditioned embarrassment. Ruby C., a working-class woman from Northern Ireland, remembers:

> Like the way they told me that when you married you had to have a man – only once – and then the Lord sent you all these kids, as many as you want. [laughs] That's what I thought!

Like Ruby C., many women recalled their lack of knowledge with humour, even though this may not have been how they experienced it at the time. Other women, though, remembered with sadness, especially when it came to talking about their own lack of fulfillment in sexual relationships. Vera W. was one of these:

> There wasn't the openness in those days. In fact, I often wish I could have my time over again. I think I should've understood it all better, sex that is. Even with my husband, whom I loved dearly, and who loved me, and who was gentleness and kindness itself, we knew very little. Before we were married I was able to talk to him and ask things and he taught me all I knew about it. He was kind and gentle, you know, and I found I could talk to him, but even then, I think we were babes in arms, both of us really. When I compare, when I think of what they know today, I think, 'Oh, fancy, if only we had known all this then, what a much happier life – married life – we could have had'. Isn't it a shame?

The prevailing view of sexuality in the first half of this century was that women did not have a sexual drive and that sex was for procreation and male pleasure only.[7] Throughout society, customs designed to preserve the modesty of women and keep predatory men at bay were observed. Mrs G., a working-class handywoman, describes one such custom prevalent at the beginning of the century:

> You went up the street in long skirts and if you had, you know, your skirt above your ankle, the chap would look at you and you'd drop your skirt. We had clips on our skirts, you see, to hold them up, but if we saw a man, we'd unclip them and let them drop. [giggles] Don't s'pose it made any difference!

It was to take several decades before Marie Stopes' revelations about women's sexual response were considered seriously by a wider audience – let alone become commonly accepted. It must be presumed that lack of knowledge about women's sexuality meant that, on the whole, neither women nor men would have had any expectations of women's potential for sexual pleasure. Several women, such as Vera W., commented that they thought that women were not as interested in sex then as they are now.

> Does this sound funny, or was it just the thing in my day. I've often wondered. I never talk about these things to people. We never had sex before marriage, never went to bed or anything like that. In five years, we never. And yet, we were quite in love with each other I'm sure. So I kept my boyfriends although I never had any sexual overtones with any of them really. Was it odd?

In a study of working-class women in north-west England from 1890–1940,[8] Elizabeth Roberts suggests that the sexual aspects of marriage did not seem to be as important to couples in those days as it grew to be in the latter part of this century. Sex was regarded as necessary for the procreation of children or as something men did for their own pleasure. Women rarely, if ever, hinted at getting any pleasure themselves from sex. Most women that we talked to had not expected to feel much sexual pleasure. Ruby C., for example, said:

> I wasn't interested in sex, like as such, you know. People then weren't because you knew nothing about it. It didn't bother you like.

It may be that modesty and a lifetime of conditioning and denial inhibited most of the women we interviewed from admitting to any expectations of sexual pleasure. Many gatherers of oral testimony have noted that even interviewees who are very open only say what they want you to know about them.

Some women did express feelings of frustration and sadness about their sexuality. Edie M. wistfully described the emptiness of her sexual life. Sex was a means of fulfilling her husband's physical needs rather than an expression of affection and closeness between them:

> When I had those four children, perhaps it only happened once, perhaps twice. So it wasn't lots of sexy nights! Never knew what love was. I'd never had no fuss made of me. Automatically happened. You went to bed and, perhaps this sort of suddenly happened and finished and away you go to sleep. No love, no care...

Lou N., a working-class woman from London, was clearly distressed not only by her lack of sexual satisfaction but also by the almost total absence of any sexual relationship at all:

> He worked behind the bar. Now, if he had any temptation it was behind the bar, wasn't it? But no, he shut up shop when I was 28. Meself I always believed that brooding on that brought on these strokes that I've had. I wouldn't have the cheek to say that to him, but I believe that. Because I was a person that had been adopted as a kid and I was living with first one person, then another, never had no settled home, I really wanted someone to make a fuss of me and all the rest of it. No, we got the kids, but, well, I had to start teasing him towards the end. I said, 'You don't only use it for one thing, you know!' The point is this: there was no affection, you know, I wasn't allowed to show it to him. But he stopped completely when I was 28. It was a terrible strain on me and I had my strokes when I was 48. And I always believed that that was the cause of it. But I think really, because we didn't know anything about sex, we were affright. That was the tension at the back of it with him and me.

Bearing in mind the social and cultural constraints and lack of knowledge already discussed, it is hard to assess how much frank discussion, if any, went on in private between women, or between women and men. Our impression is that there was very little. Lou N. summed up the situation thus:

> Well, we were all green. I was as green as that bloody chair when I got married. I was still as green when my husband died, and we'd been married 49 years! Me and Charlie, we were both green.

Hannah H. came from a middle-class background, very different from that of Lou N., but she echoed similar thoughts on the general lack of knowledge:

> I was very innocent, I was, really. There were lots of things we never really understood. I never knew what a period was until it happened to me. Used to hear girls whispering together, and shutting up when you got near, but I – I was never – never inquisitive enough. So I never knew a lot of things, really. I still don't either!

As sex was not discussed at home, children learnt about the 'facts of life' in the playground. Like Hannah H., many girls started menstruating knowing nothing about the process. Lou N. recalls:

> When I first started me periods when I was 14, I came home from school and I told the old lady what happened. 'Oh', she said, 'That's nice! But you mustn't play with boys'. And I thought it meant that you couldn't go out and play in the street with 'em. She didn't tell me no more and that's as much as I knew.

Knowledge about pregnancy and birth

> I never dreamt it would of come from there!

The fear of pregnancy may well have dampened women's sexual appetites, particularly those who had already given birth. However, many women we interviewed said that their first pregnancy and childbirth came as a total shock. It was apparent that lack of knowledge made the whole experience of birth a nightmare. Edie M. remembered with anguish her first labour:

> I remember at the very last minute I suddenly realised where it was coming from. It shook me. I was so shocked. No, I didn't know before. I don't know what I thought. But suddenly, knowing that this child would have to come out of there. I knew the size of a... Oh, I was so shocked and frightened. I said, 'Please, please, can you stop it coming out? I don't mind what pain I have. I'll suffer any pain but please can you stop it coming out?' That first one, I'd have given even me life to stop that child coming! I never dreamt it would have come from there. The very idea of your body opening like that! It's imposible! You can understand people that don't want them.

Like Edie, many women described the horror of 'not knowing where the baby was going to come out'. Mrs G., who worked as a handywoman in south-east London, confirmed that this lack of knowledge was common:

> They didn't know where it was going to come out. But they knew where it went in, didn't they? Well, it's got to come out the same place. But they're so dense some of them. I think some of them think it comes out in a bladder, like a balloon, or through the belly button. They think their

> belly opens. I said, 'It won't come out through there'. And they soon found out that it wouldn't!
>
> Well, yes, I s'pose it was frightening for the first one. You can understand it really. I used to say, 'Don't be frightened. If you're frightened, don't think that you're going to split in half, 'cause you won't'.

With virtually no antenatal classes and few books with relevant factual information for prospective parents, it is not surprising that many women had no idea how the baby was growing inside them or how it would be born. Pregnancy was not seen as something to be proud of. In fact it was often hidden, as Molly B. explains:

> Up there [South Shields] you didn't tell anyone you were pregnant till you were actually having it. You didn't discuss whether you were pregnant or not. That was a terrible thing! Even for married women it was considered shameful. After all, it showed what you'd been doing, didn't it! [laughs] They used to say, 'She's gone to bed', and you knew she was in labour. They never said, 'She's having a baby'.

While we found that all women seemed to share the same lack of knowledge, their approaches to obtaining information differed. Working-class women tended to go to their friends and sisters for facts and advice, whereas middle-class women like Vera W. chose to consult the few books that were available:

> I didn't know anything at all except I bought a book. And my doctor said, 'Throw that on the fire!' But I didn't because I was so ignorant, you see.

The midwives were very aware of how little most women knew and, like Edie B, were mostly sympathetic:

> There were no antenatal classes in my day. They didn't know anything apart from what their mothers told them, which was practically nil. They didn't know what to expect. They weren't prepared for all the pain. They weren't even told it was painful. Poor little things, they didn't know a thing. I used to go to bed and cry... Poor girls.

Even some of the midwives admitted their own initial ignorance about the 'facts of life'. Nellie H. described a situation that arose at the beginning of her nurse training where she had as little relevant or useful knowledge as the mother herself:

This story will make you laugh! It was about 1924. I was on
night duty and we always had to open the door at night.
There were no porters or anything like that. I went to the
door and there was these two ambulancemen looking
scared out of their wits.

And they said to me, 'This girl's ever so ill. Where shall
we take her?' So I said, 'Well, it depends what the matter
is with her'. So he said, 'Well, she says she's not going to
have a baby, but we think she is...'

So I said, 'Ooh, we'd better ring Sister upstairs'. So Sister
Cramp came down and she said, 'Ridiculous! You must
know you're going to have a baby. Don't be so silly girl!'
(She had got a tummy out here anyway.)

So the girl said, 'Well, I don't know anything about it, I
don't know when it happened, I don't know anything
about it'. So Sister said, 'Oh well, never mind my dear, come
on upstairs'.

So they carried her up the three flights of stairs –
everything was jolly hard work in those days – and then
Sister said to me, 'Well, you'd better keep an eye on her
while I go and see all about her'.

I stayed with this girl, so I said, 'What's your name dear?'
So she said, 'Venus'. (Crikey, what a name!)

So I said, 'Oh well, Sister says you're going to have a baby'.
She said, 'Well, I don't know anything about it'. So I said,
'Well you must do, surely?' Though I myself didn't know
much about it because, you know, in those days our parents
never used to tell us. And when I went into hospital,
honest to goodness I had no idea where a baby came from.
I was 21. I had no idea where a baby came from or how it
got there, or anything! I mean, I just thought they came!
So, I thought, 'I s'pose she's the same.'

Any rate, Sister came back and she said, 'Well, I'll show
you what to do to get her ready to have her baby'. Well, in
the meantime this girl had said to me, 'I really don't know
anything about it'. So I said, 'Well, I don't know dear, it's
no good telling me because if Sister says you're going to have
a baby, you are'.

She said, 'Well, I really don't know anything about it'.
So she was crying and carrying on you know, like anything.
I suppose it was when she had a pain but I didn't realise
then. She said, 'Oh dear, Oh dear, I don't know what I'm
going to do...' So I said, 'Well, just keep calm. There's no

good shouting'. I said, 'You'll be all right in a minute, dear. Sister will be looking after you'.

Sister came back and Venus had the baby and it was a lovely baby. It's interesting because when I saw that baby coming, I really couldn't believe it. You know, I thought, 'Oooh, I wonder how it comes out of there...?'

So then she said, 'I want to see John...' So Sister said, 'Well, who's John?' She said, 'We live on a barge, you see, on the Thames, and these people live on the barge next to me'. Well, then we found out that John was the father of the baby. But I don't think either of them really knew what had happened. I really don't, because they were so innocent. I s'pose they had...you know...been...together and...done...what they wanted to do...but they didn't realise it...that they were going to have a baby. They really didn't. She was only young. She was about 18, I think.

Anyway, she confessed to Sister afterwards that she had something to do with this young man because she said, 'He's nice and we like one another. My mother used to grumble and say I shouldn't go over there to the other barge but I liked going over there to see him'. So I s'pose that was real love, wasn't it? I've never had real...well, I did really. I had a young man but he was killed in the First World War. He was only 19 and I was 18 so I didn't want to get married then. I was quite happy not to...

So that was the first baby I saw being born and I was ever so interested. But I couldn't work out how it got there even then! When I think of how daft I was! I really was silly, you know! But then, if you don't really know about men and boys at the time, well, then you don't really know, do you? Well, at the time I thought that they must have just been kissing and cuddling. Well, that's OK. I don't see how that's going to bring a baby! It was real funny. By the time I started to do my midwifery training I'd woke up a bit!

During the first half of this century midwives may have gained access to information about 'the facts of life' through their training, but the vast majority of women suffered from an extreme lack of knowledge and dire level of misinformation. It caused difficulties in their sex lives and pregnancies, and also had major repercussions for women trying to control their fertility.

References

1. Jordan,Terry, *Agony Columns*, MacDonald Optima, London, 1988, Chapter 5.
2. *ibid*, pp.100–101.
3. Arbuthnot Lane, Sir W. (ed.), *The Modern Woman's Home Doctor*, Odhams Press Ltd., London, 1930s (not dated), pp.120–145
4. Stopes, Marie, *Married Love*, G.P. Putnam & Sons, London, 1918.
5. *ibid*, p.63.
6. *ibid*, p.28.
7. Lewis, Jane, *Women in England 1870–1950*, Wheatsheaf Books, Sussex, 1984.
8. Roberts, Elizabeth, *A Woman's Place – An Oral History of Working-class Women: 1890–1940*, Basil Blackwell, Oxford, 1984.

5 Birth control

> You just took what come, didn't ya? Just took a chance,
> didn't ya?

If most women knew little about sex, they knew even less about
contraception. Couples who wanted to limit the size of their
families had difficulty finding out how to do so. In the 1920s and
1930s, there was little effective and safe birth control provision
for working-class women. The first birth control clinics, such as
the Marie Stopes clinics, were set up by voluntary organisations
in the 1920s, but there were no state-run clinics until 1931.

Mabel P. trained as a midwife in 1912, having been refused entry
to medical school. Eventually, she managed to train as a doctor
and worked as an obstetrician and gynaecologist for the rest of her
professional life. She described how she helped set up a birth
control clinic to alleviate some of the hardship caused by repeated
pregnancies. She had witnessed the problems while working as a
district midwife in Somerset:

> In Bristol we started up a birth control clinic for the poor
> women in Bedminster, and the city took it over once it was
> working well. Mainly, we fitted caps there. It was a very poor
> area.

Outside of the clinics, few family doctors saw it as part of their
job to give advice on birth control, and they were often discouraged from doing so by both medical training schools and their professional bodies.[1] The bulk of medical opinion was opposed to birth
control in the 1920s, as this extract from a letter by a distinguished
female gynaecologist to the *British Medical Journal* shows:

> The people and nations who practise artificial prevention
> of conception and who therefore have no restraint in their
> sexual passions are likely to become effeminate and
> degenerate. The removal of the sanction of matrimony
> and the unhindered and unbalanced sexual indulgence

that would follow would war against self-control, chivalry
and self-respect.[2]

According to handywoman Mrs G. (who tended to be somewhat
disparaging about doctors), working-class women did not consider
turning to their family doctor for help with birth control. She
laughed heartily when she commented:

> What's the good of going to the doctor? He could only put
> another one in there couldn't he?!

Birth control became part of the political agenda in the 1920s
when women in the Labour Party fought hard to get their party
to support birth control provision. They were to be disappointed
though. In 1924, the newly elected first Labour government
refused to accept state responsibility for such services.

Battles around the issue of birth control continued throughout
the 1920s and 1930s. Much of the resistance to contraception was
on moral grounds. Contraception was seen as a temptation to
promiscuity. In the 1930s, such concerns were summarised in the
handbook, *The Modern Woman's Home Doctor*. A chapter entitled,
'The Modern Practice of Birth Control', begins:

> The harm that might possibly be done by giving people the
> knowledge of how to control conception can be summed
> up under three headings – namely, sexual excess, intercourse
> between those who are unmarried, and an increase in the
> number of those who are childless.[3]

Edie M., a working-class London woman, remembers the
prevailing attitude that assumed contraception was for use only
in extra-marital relationships:

> See, I mean, we never knew how not to have 'em. Besides,
> a respectable husband wouldn't have thought of using a
> French letter with his wife. Only I s'pose with outside
> women he might have done. But they were never
> mentioned inside a marriage – working-class married homes
> anyway.

Marie Stopes did much to initiate changes in attitudes towards
contraception by setting birth control within the context of
marriage, thereby rendering it more respectable. In 1926, she
published a series of articles in the popular magazine, *John Bull*,
which elicited over 20,000 requests for abortion information
alone![4]

The philosophy behind fertility control, however, was not necessarily altruistic. Marie Stopes, for example, was a eugenicist. Her interest was in curbing the breeding of the working classes so that the British race would be of 'better stock'. June Rose, who has recently researched the life of Marie Stopes comments:

> Marie *was* a radical, but she was a right-wing radical... Her birth control clinics were set up to alleviate the burden of working-class women who otherwise were destined to have large families bred in extreme poverty. But one shouldn't lose sight of her motives – the creation and preservation of a system of breeding which is in many respects similar to that advocated in Nazi Germany.[5]

After the First World War, there was a great fear that contraception could lead to a devastating depletion in the numbers of the British race available to defend the Empire:

> Those who have as many enemies as the British Empire must for their own safety have plenty of children and meet those enemies at the gate. [Quote from a judge in 1920 when sentencing a professional abortionist.[6]]

With the reduction in population following the First World War, there was great emphasis on 're-building the nation' so women were encouraged to have more children – not fewer. In women's magazines of the inter-war period, there were often references to the patriotic role of mothers. In a *Woman's Own* article, 'Building an A1 Nation', Nurse Vincent proclaims:

> A healthy mother produces a healthy baby and the mothers of the Nation must be kept in A1 condition if we are to have A1 children.[7]

In 1930, the government partially gave way on the issue of birth control by allowing existing maternity and child welfare clinics to give advice on preventing pregnancy to expectant and nursing mothers whose health would be injured by further pregnancies.

Four years later, in 1934, local authorities and regional health boards were given the power to set up birth control clinics or assist voluntary organisations in so doing. However, this was not compulsory. Provision varied from area to area, as indeed it does today. There was still much opposition to initiating birth control provision, and outside the cities, clinics were non-existent.

Despite the opposition, the number of clinics increased from less than 20 in the period 1921–1931 to about 60 in the period 1931–1941. By 1951, there were approximately 140 clinics offering birth control advice. However, these clinics only gave information and advice to married women or those who could prove that they were engaged to be married – a policy still in existence when the authors were teenagers in the 1960s.

None of the women we interviewed had attended such a clinic, and only one middle-class woman had used contraception:

> When I'd been married about six months and got used to married life, I said, 'Oh we won't bother any more now with precautions, I'm ready to have a child'. He wasn't a bit willing really. He was going to be jealous, of course. And then he said to me, 'Well, I don't mind as long as he doesn't come before me'.

This account is in vivid contrast to the testimony of the working-class women, most of whom had a more fatalistic attitude to childbearing, and indeed to life. As Edie M. says:

> And that was the time we was having babies all the time. Just get looked at and you got a baby. Well, there were FLs [French letters] about, I suppose, but they was never spoken of. I never used nothing. You just took what come, didn't ya? Just took a chance, didn't ya?

Molly B., who grew up in South Shields, Tyneside, describes the devastating effect that constant childbearing had on everyone's lives:

> My mother was one of 21 children. She was 17 when she married in 1914. She had her first baby a year later and in all she had eight of us. Three died in infancy and two were killed in the war. I remember her saying, 'I wouldn't have had the children if I'd known what I know now. No way would it have happened. I didn't want a lot of children but there was no birth control then'. So many of the children died because of the terrible conditions and I think death and poverty and hunger were just accepted. When a child died it was another mouth you didn't have to feed. There was no room for being sentimental. But then, as soon as you finished breast-feeding one baby, another would be on its way...and so it went on.

While breast-feeding can afford women a certain degree of protection from pregnancy – if they consistently and frequently feed the baby on demand – it has never been a reliable form of contraception. Elsie B., who was a district midwife in rural Devon all her working life, starting in 1929, remembers women trying to control their fertility in this way:

> You'd got an old idea that while the mother was breast-feeding her baby she wouldn't become pregnant. So some of them used to feed for a long time. You see, there wasn't much birth control around in those days.

Even when women managed to get to a birth control clinic, there could still be problems. Lou N. describes her friend's experience of going to a clinic in wartime rural England:

> When I was evacuated away, there was a woman there who told me this story. Her husband come on leave – this is true – and she kept on having babies very quick. She didn't want no more children so she goes to the clinic. Apparently, in those days, they used a thing called a 'Rendell' [a spermicide pessary containing quinine]. It looks like a half of a Brazil nut. One of the women at the clinic said, 'Oh, I tell you what Bessie, you meet me on Tuesday and I'll give you something'. See, well, she gave 'em these Rendells but she didn't tell her what she was to do with 'em. You can guess what happened, can't you? Well, she goes up to bed about five or ten minutes before her husband and she hadn't been up there five minutes and she's screaming blue murder. Ugh! Choking! She'd put it in her mouth instead of anywhere else!
>
> We tried the French letters once, y' know. My husband's brother gave him one, and again, with no instructions. And of course me and him, being green, knew nothing about sizes. Oh, he nearly went barmy. Never again! So bang went that idea! It was far too small.

Given the evidence about the lack of use of contraception, it is surprising that statistics show a steady decline in average family size since the beginning of the 20th century. On average, a married couple in mid-Victorian England would have 5.5 to six live births, whereas the statistic for a couple in the period 1925–1929 was 2.2 live births.[8]

Family size figures suggest that many couples used some kind of 'unofficial' birth control. Deirdre Beddoe suggests that possible methods used were restraint, abstinence and the 'safe period'.[9] We would add abortion and withdrawal to this list. When women referred to their husbands' 'taking care' of them or 'being careful', they were often using popular euphemisms for the withdrawal method. In some cases, the phrase 'taking care of me' may have implied abstinence and restraint, the idea being that 'decent' men control themselves and do not expect 'it' too often.

In her article, 'Married Life and Birth Control between the Wars',[10] Diana Gittins questions the theory that the decrease in the birth rate for married couples in the 1920s can be attributed to economic influences or the availability of improved contraception since these came much later. She considers changes in attitude to family size to be crucially important, and this is usually connected to the couple's increased expectations for their standard of living. She also found that use of contraception was related to the woman's occupation prior to marriage. Those who worked outside of the home were more likely to want to limit their family. They were also more likely to know how to do this. This was borne out by evidence given to us during the interviews.

Apart from abortions, the only forms of contraception available in the first half of this century were barrier methods. The Marie Stopes clinics favoured the use of the cervical cap in conjunction with a jelly or pessary. After the 1940s, the diaphragm or 'Dutch cap' became increasingly popular. Centuries-old barrier methods, such as sponges soaked in solutions of quinine, oil, lemon juice or vinegar, were in use and may well have had some spermicidal value.

The use of birth control methods such as the diaphragm, cervical cap or greasy spermicidal pessaries could be problematic in homes where there was no inside toilet or running water, or where family members had to share bedrooms. Perhaps for this reason, the women we interviewed only ever mentioned using condoms, which they referred to as 'French letters'.

Sterilization was rare, but one middle-class woman, Vera W., was sterilized for medical reasons:

> Incidentally, they sterilized me at the same time as I had the Caesarean – tied off my tubes – because they said that I shouldn't have any more children. So they got my husband's permission and sterilized me. I didn't mind at all. I'd got one child and actually my husband, he didn't particularly want children. That was my doing, my wanting.

According to the midwives we interviewed, it was not women's modesty that prevented them from discussing contraceptive methods. Rather, they had a general lack of information. Even midwifery textbooks of the time made no mention of contraception, and midwives generally felt that they had little to offer in terms of helping women to control their fertility. As Edith B. said:

> There wasn't much family planning available then. I think it came on the man's side. They never asked me for advice. No, no. It was a forbidden subject. Nothing about anything like that. My mother never told me about a thing. Nothing. I mean, I thought I was dying when...I was about 15...'Oh ma, I'm dying, bleeding to death!' She'd told me nothing at all. I hope if you ever have a girl you'll tell her; or even a boy. They should know too.

Elizabeth C. was a district midwife in Battersea, south-west London, for many years before and after the NHS was set up in 1948. Known as 'Aunty Betty' to her clients, she was unusual in that she felt able to give useful advice about birth control.

> Yes, they did ask me how to prevent having babies. They did have condoms and the cap. They went to the doctor for those, but I knew a certain amount about the 'safe period'.

Elizabeth C. was the only interviewee who mentioned the 'safe period'. Possibly she was remembering a later time in her midwifery career, since it is questionable how much accurate information about the 'safe period' was available before the mid-1930s. In the 1920s, midwives were taught that conception was most likely to occur around the time of menstruation. Birth control clinics were giving the same misinformation as midwifery textbooks, such as Fairbairn's *Textbook for Midwives*:

> Though it has never been proved, it is probable that ovulation and menstruation occur together, and in any case it is quite certain that there is a very close connection between the two.[11]

In 1930, researchers Ogino in Japan and Knaus in Austria independently determined that ovulation occurred mid-cycle.[12] Over the next decade this information filtered through to the midwifery textbooks.

It was not until the 1960s that midwifery textbooks contained a section on contraception. In the 1920s and 1930s midwives were actively discouraged from giving advice about contraception. A directive in the May 1934 edition of *Nursing Notes* reflects this:

> Advice on the question of contraceptives does not come within the practice or work of a midwife as such; if for health reasons she thinks there is a risk in her patient again becoming pregnant, she should refer her to her doctor or a clinic for medical examination and advice: as the training she received as a midwife does not give her the necessary knowledge to judge whether or not if for medical reasons it is necessary for her patient to use contraceptives...

There was also concern about the conclusions that could be drawn if midwives were involved in distributing contraceptives:

> There is a danger of them being falsely accused of being abortionists.[13]

Midwives may have been anxious to distance themselves from the issue of abortion, but for many of the women in their care, abortion was the main form of fertility control. Whenever we asked working-class women about birth control, they always mentioned abortion. While almost all of them had never used contraception, they all knew how to procure an abortion. Several described giving themselves abortions. This led us to conclude that for many women, abortion was one of the most common forms of birth control.

References

1. Holdsworth, Angela, *Out of the Dolls House*, BBC Books, 1988, p.96.
2. Cited in Hall, Ruth (ed.), *Dear Dr. Stopes – Sex in the 1920s*, Penguin, London, 1978, p.81.
3. Arbuthnot Lane, Sir W. (ed.), *The Married Woman's Home Doctor*, Odhams Press Ltd., London, 1930s, p.94.
4. Hall, Ruth (ed.), *Dear Dr. Stopes – Sex in the 1920s*, Penguin, London, 1978, p.12.
5. McCrystal, Cal, 'The Monster and the Master Race', *The Independent on Sunday*, 23 August, 1992.

6. Kenner, Charmian, *No Time For Women: Exploring Women's Health in the 1930s and Today*, Pandora Press, London, 1985, p.42.
7. *Woman's Own*, 7 July 1934.
8. Beddoe, Deirdre, *Discovering Women's History*, Pandora Press, London, 1983, p.182.
9. *ibid*, p.180.
10. Gittins, Diana, 'Married Life and Birth Control between the Wars', *Oral History – The Journal of the Oral History Society*, vol 3, no. 2, autumn 1975, pp.53–64.
11. Fairbairn, John S, *A Textbook for Midwives*, 4th edition, Oxford University Press, 1924, p.48.
12. Robertson, William H, *An Illustrated History of Contraception*, The Parthenon Publishing Group, Carnforth, Lancs, 1990, p.118.
13. *Nursing Notes*, May 1934, p.69.

6 Abortion: 'there was no other way'

> That was the first thing I knew how to...not prevent, but how to get rid of... There was no other way.

Here, Edie M. describes how it felt to be a working-class woman in the 1920s and '30s. Unless a woman wanted and could support a large family, her fertility must have felt like a huge burden. More babies meant more mouths to feed, more work to do and increasing poverty. As soon as one baby was weaned, another was on its way, and in pre-NHS days it was extremely difficult to find out about contraception. There were few clinics and most GPs refused to give advice. So how did women control their fertility? Withdrawal, abstinence and plain avoidance all depended on the man's co-operation, so for many women abortion was the only viable option.

Abortion was declared illegal in 1803. In the 1930s and '40s, it became legal only in exceptional circumstances – to save the life of the woman. The situation persisted until the 1967 Abortion Act legalised abortion.

In the decades before 1967, there were many campaigners – including members of the Women's Co-operative Guild and the Abortion Law Reform Association – who wanted to legalise abortion. The latter was strongly supported by feminists such as Stella Browne and Dora Russell, who argued that a change in the law was necessary because so many women died each year as a result of illegal abortions. In 1934, for instance, 13 per cent of maternal deaths resulted from abortions. They were mostly of married women, and most resulted from infection.

Before abortions were legalised, the birth control clinics could offer no help to women seeking abortions. Women had to arrange them themselves, and they could die from the various complications that could arise from abortion: shock, haemorrhage or infection. Instruments were usually not sterile; the uterus could be perforated; the contents might not be wholly removed. Women could also suffer from resulting sterility, pelvic inflammation or miscarriage in subsequent pregnancies.

As well as using instruments, women also took pills and various herbal concoctions in an attempt to abort pregnancies. It is impossible to quantify the long-term effects on their health. Concoctions containing poisonous substances such as lead would, at the very least, have had a debilitating effect. In the worst cases, they would have proved fatal.

It should be remembered that the women we interviewed usually talked as though contraception and abortion were the same thing. Women did not define abortion in the way we do now. It was seen as a form of birth control. This was discussed in the midwifery journal, *Nursing Notes*, in January 1928:

> There is one matter that some midwives and nurses may not have realised and which adds a complication when dealing with uneducated persons viz. the difficulty in making them understand the very great difference between contraception and procuring abortion. Midwives know very well how common the latter has become since the economic and housing difficulty has been so acute, and should not forget how the two questions are often confused.[1]

Several of the women we interviewed had given themselves abortions, often more than once. Nearly all of them knew how to 'get rid of a baby' should the need arise. As Edie M. says:

> My sister was a very boyish type of girl, very...well, never talked about sex or men or nothing. She was...how can I say it...very down to earth. Me and my sister never talked sex. But one day she was telling me she found out how to get rid of babies. When she told me, it was the first time we'd ever talked sex in our lives; grew up together, worked together, lived together, but never really talked until then when she told me how to do it.
>
> Soap and water injection – you used to make the solution of soapy water, best yellow soap, you have to have a pure soap, not any old soap; it had to be a pure baby soap. You'd get the syringe and put it inside you. She said, 'You can feel your womb inside, don't press inside, just put the nozzle to your womb and get the soapy water to it'. I put myself in hospital twice with bad haemorrhages after doing that.

The method Edie described would have been in common usage in the 1920s and 1930s and would have been more effective in causing an abortion than most of the concoctions taken orally. Molly B. and her sister Lily N. remember:

> Oh yes, there was back street goings on. Because, don't forget, South Shields is a port and a lot of seamen came in and there was a lot of prostitutes down by the docks, thousands of 'em. And there was a chemist down there where all these 'awful women' – as my mum referred to them – went to get pills and potions to make them abort. I don't know what they used. Someone told me they used cotton wool dipped in some strong disinfectant to put up inside them, but they also used knitting needles and crochet hooks as well. (*Lily*)
>
> Oh no, it wasn't just the prostitutes. I think married women did something too. Hardly anyone had any work for a start. Awful wasn't it, Lil? And they just couldn't afford to have anymore. I think women got quite desperate about all the children. I quite think that women hated sex up there, the majority of them, because they were frightened to have another baby. (*Molly*)

Since it was impossible to quantify an illegal practice that people were at pains to deny, the abortion statistics of the time may well have been a gross underestimation of a common practice. Nevertheless, they make salutory reading. In 1938, a government committee on abortion estimated that at least 90,000 illegal abortions were performed every year,[2] and the 1937 *Report on an Investigation into Maternity Mortality* observed that the rate of criminal abortion nearly doubled between the years 1911–1920 and 1930–1933.[3]

Although none of the women we interviewed had been to an abortionist, most knew of their existence. Lou N. told us:

> When I was a child I ear-wagged and apparently a woman across the road – Mrs Thackery – apparently she used to do jobs with a crochet hook – it sounded terrible to me but I do remember that.

The decision to abort usually seemed to be made by the woman. In fact, abortion was one of the few controls that women had over their bodies. Ruby C., however, was given abortion-inducing tablets by her mother, and later by her husband, without her full knowledge or consent.

> My mother gave me these tablets. As a matter of fact, I never even knew what they were. Mother says, 'You have to take these to help you'. I thought they were just to – you know, boost you up like a kind of tonic or something! I didn't know I was losing the baby. I got up and oh, I was flooding all over, on my dress, on the chair and my mother hurried my friend out, and then my mother said, 'Oh, that's good'. That was all I knew about it. I just felt light-headed and all, like that.

Ruby also recalled another occasion that made her suspicious:

> There was another time when my husband brought me some tablets. I had an idea what they were. I was out at the pictures and he had give me these – 'sweets' he called them. We were coming home down an alleyway and I said 'Oh, I don't know what's wrong, whether I want to go to the toilet', and I had a miscarriage down an alleyway. Oh God. I thought nothing of it, 'cause I didn't know anything and it just didn't worry me 'cause when you don't know... it's silly.

Abortions were very often described as miscarriages. When we started interviewing, we probably missed several accounts of abortion because we assumed that 'miscarriage' meant an accidental rather than conscious termination of the pregnancy. For example, Edie M. initially talked about her miscarriages, but later redefined them as abortions. The women's stories show that abortion was seen as a normal event – one more hazard of being a woman. Significantly, Edie continued:

> I worked half my young life with haemorrhages. Now I know that it could have been ever so dangerous, but then you just got up and went to work, go out to the toilet...I was always in a state of haemorrhage. I never knew anything else and I'm sure all the people I knew never did. I caused a bad illness over it. I used to get pregnant very, very easily. That first marriage, there wasn't much sex in it at all. Perhaps twice a week if that, and there you are, suddenly you're pregnant and not even a love affair.

However, when we discussed abortion with Lou N., she said she didn't know of any woman who were aborting themselves:

Except this woman was having a baby and she had to get
rid of it because her two children were over 20 or so, a good
age, and they were so disgusted with their own mother that
the poor devil had bought herself a lace corset and she got
someone to pull it as tight as possible every day, and that's
how she killed the baby. That's the only thing I ever
remember.

When we rephrased the question as: 'You didn't hear of
anything you could take to help you bring on a period if you were
a bit late, or...?' she replied:

No...unless you took Beecham's pills...that's the only thing
I remember they had. So whenever I thought I was...that's
what I took, because I didn't believe in a lot of medicine,
see. But I did do that, just in case.

In fact, Lou N. was regularly taking something in an attempt
to terminate a possible pregnancy, but she certainly did not
define this as an abortion. The women we talked to mostly sym-
pathised with other women who found themselves driven to
abortion rather than face yet another pregnancy and child to raise.
Abortion was seen as an awful thing to have to do, but to the
mother, not to the foetus.

Edie M., however, did have misgivings about what she had done:

I must've done one in Leadenhall market. I had one when
I was working in a kitchen there. It was through using the
syringe. That baby must've been quite far on. The barmaid
that picked it up and put it down the toilet, she said, 'It was
fully formed, Edie, it was'. She said she'd put her black apron
over it – they used to wear black aprons, barmaids – and put
it in the toilet. I had a job to get home. I had a big haemorrhage at the City – I had to go down to the ladies toilet.
    My brain – (I think) – Oh, God – I had to push it out, like
I do my daughter's death, I had to push it away, cos you'd
never live if you thought of what you done.

She also remembers the hospital staff's attitude to abortion:

And the hospitals weren't very kind to you. They're not
today either, they don't like abortions. 'Did you do
anything?' You tell a lie up to your teeth. 'No, I've never
done anything'.

Ivy D. remembers telling lies when she had an abortion in the 1930s to protect the woman who helped her:

> It was a really secret thing. The woman who came and did it said, 'Don't tell anyone what you've had done or who did it'. I promised that and I never let her down. I didn't even tell my husband. They all thought it was a natural miscarriage.
>
> I don't know where the woman lived. She came to my home. I don't know who she was really. A friend told me about her. It was all very secret. She knew she'd get into trouble if she got found out. She was just a local woman – well-known in the area for what she did – who helped women out. She didn't ask for payment but I just gave her what I'd got. I was so anxious to get her out of the house really. I used to save the rent in those days in a little cup beside my bed and I just tipped it out into her hand. I was really frightened, you know.
>
> I didn't really want to have an abortion but my husband didn't want us to be confined to the house again. You see, we used to go out a lot before we had the children. We'd had two babies already. One cried all the time and we wasn't very well off in those days. He said, 'Oh no, we're going to be confined for another five years – another crying baby'. He was a kind man but he just didn't want another baby. It was awful, really. When you're pregnant everything's enlarged, isn't it. Everything feels worse than it is. He didn't know what I was doing, but I tried everything. Pills, gin...and none of it worked. So I was four and a half months gone. It was too long really, wasn't it. It was too late. When I had the next one, I had a terrible labour, had to have forceps in the end. That was punishment for the abortion, that was...
>
> She came to my home and she did it with needles. She put needles up inside me. And I was in agony all day. Of course, the woman what done it had gone. As soon as she did it, she went. It's wicked, really. It's cruel, isn't it. It was a long labour. They called the lady doctor out. And I remember this doctor kept looking at herself in my full-length mirror in the bedroom because she was very glamorous, only young. I'll always remember that bit.
>
> I lost the baby in the chamber. I saw it, you know. They would never have allowed that in hospital, would they? I can see it now, you know. It was a little girl. The eyes were

shut and all bluey. I'll always remember that. And its little
arms all folded up... It was very upsetting. I don't know
what they did with her body.

I had to go in hospital. The doctor at home, she thought
it was a natural one but she said, 'You'll have to go in. It's
an incomplete abortion'. I was haemorrhaging. I nearly died.
It was really frightening. And the doctor in hospital said to
me, 'You've been interfered with. This isn't an ordinary
abortion'. I said, 'Beechams pills', kept saying, 'Beechams
pills'. That's all I said. So I kept her secret. I never let her
down. But they were horrible to me in there...

Jane W. remembers similar attitudes from hospital staff:

When I was in hospital a long time they put them down
the other end of the ward. They'd call them 'the naughty
ward'. There was one woman next to me. She used to talk
to me, and what she didn't get up to was nobody's business!
She used to go out with other men. When she was pregnant,
what she used to do...well, she'd have different things
done to her. Oh, I used to be shocked. The things I used to
hear in there. And that's dangerous what they'd do. They
gamble with their lives. They can take it, you know, get
away with it. But it's silly of them. I mean, gamble on my
life? – no way.

We met only one woman who had been offered an abortion by
a doctor. It was Vera W. It was unclear whether the doctor
considered her life to be at risk from continuing the pregnancy
(she was a small woman with a large baby) or whether it was an
option because she was middle-class and able to pay. Either way,
it would have been a very late abortion, presumably carried out
by abdominal surgery:

I was about five foot then and he was eight and three
quarter pounds born. He was very large. I carried him – right,
way up here. So – they told me that all the bits of my inside
were pushed to my back, as the baby made room for
himself, and the last two months I used to faint about the
house. In fact, at seven months Dr M. said that – um – I
could still have the baby taken away if I wished. But I
wanted very badly to have a child and I had a feeling that
it was going to be the only one.

Some women knowingly risked their lives time and again by giving themselves abortions rather than increasing their poverty with another child. It was not just a question of 'another mouth to feed'. Another baby could make it impossible for the mother to earn the only income in the family. Edie M. explained this to us and described with great sadness the mental and physical threat posed by the trap in which she found herself:

> Once, I'd done the soapy water in the morning and the mis-carriage started to happen on the tram on the way to work. I could feel something happening on the tram. So just as I was going on the platform to go in the lift at Charing Cross, this miscarriage started, so I crouched down by the way and I covered me face. Two ladies came; one had an ear trumpet and the other must have been her maid or something. She said, 'Anything wrong?' I said, 'Yes, please help me. I've got a haemorrhage. I think I've miscarried'. So they got a porter. I was taken up in the lift and a sacking canvas thing with poles was put round. I don't know where they got it from. I had me face covered up all the time in case anyone knew me – I wasn't known there, of course, but I'd been travelling regularly from Hammersmith to Stockwell – and I was taken away to St. Giles Hospital. I was kept there a few days and then went back to work, where I had another big haemorrhage! There was a wonderful mistress there and she brought miles of tablecloth to help me. So I was taken back to hospital.
>
> We were in dire poverty then and we owed half a week's rent. I'd told the landlady – loaded with rings and diamonds, she was – that we would be moving out to my sister's in Dulwich as soon as I was well enough. I'd had ten haem-orrhages in a week and my bed was tipped up – you can guess how ill I was. And she only put the bailiff in! I couldn't get over it 'cause it wasn't a lot of rent we owed. 'If you like', he said, 'You can call your doctor in and I won't be able to touch the place if you can't be moved'. 'Well, I mustn't be moved but we're going up my sister's 'cause we can't afford to stay here'. (Twenty-five shillings – and me not working, two children and only Alec's dole – there was no way we could stay.) So I made arrangements to go to my sister's on the Friday. Took the home up there on a barrow – he pushed the barrow from Brixton up to the top of Dulwich with our home on it. I had to wait in the bed 'til my sister finished work. She came with Dolly who was

courting my cousin, to fetch me. They helped me dress in
the bed and then they helped me to a tram, both holding
an arm each side. I was all right 'til I got up to Braemar Road,
up the top of Dog Kennel Hill, and as I got off the tram
there, I haemorrhaged. So my sister picked me up in her
arms and ran me quick down the street to her house. I was
put in her front room, bed tipped again, and the doctor was
sent for.

I always say that people should be very careful when they
speak in front of unconscious people 'cause nine times
out of ten they can hear. I heard every word what was said.
I kept sinking down into a black hole – that's the only way
I can describe it – a black hole. I kept sinking down. But I
heard the doctor say, 'Send for an ambulance', and I heard
the ambulancemen say, 'We can't move her, she's got no
pulse. We'll come back in the morning'. I heard the doctor
say, 'Well I'll come back every hour'. Yes, I was very ill. It's
happened on about four or five occasions in my life.

See, girls today fall deeply in love and you think, 'Poor
devil', but in those days you was just going to work to bring
in some food. That's why today I think I'm a much harder
person. I used to be a romantic young thing but this old
memory don't shut much out either. It goes over the worst
parts. Sometimes I have to block it out and think 'Well, let's
think of some nice things'. You can't live with some of the
things you've done...

Midwives and abortion

The midwives we met varied in both their memories of abortion
and their attitudes towards it. Some, like Nellie H, denied ever
having come across it:

No, I didn't know of it. I don't remember any.

Others spoke about abortion as an inevitable part of women's
lives:

There used to be the old slippery elm. And some used to use
the crochet hook that went into the uterus. Some of the
mothers died, you know. Oh yes, the slippery elm was
round the corner – there was a woman who was doing it.
And the poor women who were at their wits' end – they'd
do anything to get rid of the foetus. (*Josephine M.*)

Midwives who had also trained as nurses often had memories of women being brought into hospital dangerously ill as a result of giving themselves abortions. Florence W. remembers that many of these women died:

> I did wonder once with my mother. She'd had a miscarriage and I remember seeing her desperately ill. I think they used to talk amongst themselves about this, but of course it didn't register until I became older and looked back on it. When I was doing general training, it first came home to me because in the women's medical ward we did have women that came in and died of septicaemia as a result of these abortions. There were no antibiotics at that time. Sulphonomides were introduced in the 1930s and if you could get to them before they got too seriously ill you could save them.

Elsie B., who had done direct-entry midwifery training, had no such memories. Like many midwives practising in the 1930s, she disassociated herself from the subject of abortion.

> I didn't meet any, but I think they were about. I don't think there was so much of it then. You had the odd miscarriage but you accepted them as inevitable, which I think most of them were.

Many midwives like Esther S., suspected that abortions took place but were not directly involved in them:

> There was an old wives' tale about using pennyroyal to get rid of their babies, and all that business. I don't think they told their midwife about trying to get rid of babies so I didn't come across a lot. So maybe there were more than I knew. But they just had big families and accepted it.

We got the impression that midwives felt that they had to keep themselves ignorant of abortion to ensure they weren't accused of being involved in an illegal activity. Such an accusation could lead to a hearing before the Plenary Board of the Central Midwives Board, followed by removal from the Register of Practising Midwives. A midwife would be an obvious person to go to for advice, so it would be important to keep her name clear.

The same line of reasoning could apply to handywomen. One of the major accusations levelled at handywomen by those who wanted to drive them out of midwifery was that they were putting women's lives at risk by performing abortions. In his thesis on handywomen, Bob Little argues that handywomen would not have risked their reputation and livelihood by acting as abortionists, too.[4] Other authors such as Mary Chamberlain, however, have assumed that the handywomen and the abortionists were one and the same person.[5]

From our research, we feel that it is extremely unlikely that handywomen were involved with abortions. The handywoman's work was primarily in attending births, looking after the mother and baby post-natally, and laying out the dead. No woman we interviewed ever made a connection between handywomen and abortion. They would often talk about 'the woman you'd go to' if you wanted an abortion, but in no cases was she 'the woman you called for' if you were having a baby or wanted someone to lay out your dead. Ivy D. confirms this:

> She didn't do midwifery or anything like that. Oh no. She just did abortions. The midwives were more honourable. My husband's mother used to lay out the dead but she certainly didn't have anything to do with abortions. That was always a different person.

So who were the abortionists? Studies by Moya Woodside and Dr J. C. Weir suggest that most abortionists were women. Most were older, married and from the lower-middle or working classes. They charged for their services but all regarded themselves as 'helping'.[6]

One of the authors of this book had a conversation with her grandparents about the various roles of members of the community in the Berkshire village where they grew up. The grandparents remembered a number of different practitioners who could advise and treat a woman. Granny Richardson was the local washerwomen and handywoman, and she delivered all the village women's babies. The barber was also a herbalist, and performed abortions. He was also used by the village people to treat illnesses when they could not afford to pay the doctor (a common occurrence). Lastly, there was the chemist, who made up special medicines for individual complaints according to his own recipes, and who also 'helped women not to have children'. It was unclear from the account what exactly 'helping a woman not to have children' involved. Again, the dividing line between contraception and abortion is very hazy in people's memories.[7]

Midwives were very aware of 'picking up the pieces' when abortion went wrong. They were sometimes called in when women were left with life-threatening haemorrhage following what was euphemistically described as 'miscarriage'. Mary W., who from the early 1930s, practised for 37 years on the district in a Yorkshire mining community, gives an example of how frightening that could be:

> Oh yes, trying to get rid of the pregnancy, that was quite common. But they wouldn't tell you. I remember once – this was before '37, the old doctor asked me if I'd go. You see in those days you couldn't get an ambulance if they'd done it (the abortion) in the middle of the night. You'd have to wait till the ambulance man came on duty at 8 o'clock next morning. He said 'Will you go and stay with this woman until we can get her into hospital tomorrow?'
>
> Doctor said, 'Of course, you know, nurse, she hasn't done anything, hasn't taken anything!...' 'Oh, I don't think about it, doctor'. But...later I had the old nerves on the go! She was practically at the last gasp. And do you know? – she recovered, that woman, and she lived to be ninety! Yes, she already had a large family. They would never tell you what they'd done – a mixture of herbs, I don't know. Gin and raspberry leaves was one thing, I think, but there was very little birth control. It was sort of a woman's mission in life to have babies. Families of six to ten were the usual thing.

Katherine L. and Margaret A., sisters who practised as domiciliary midwives in Essex for 28 years, starting in the late '30s, talked about keeping a tactful distance from the local woman who performed abortions. Katherine explained:

> You heard things. There was one woman here in the town who had a name for it – but they could never catch her. But they knew she existed. They knew her and I s'pose you could call it a brothel. I don't know whether she did have a brothel. I wouldn't be surprised. But she could perform abortions on pregnant girls. I wouldn't know how she did it. I mean, we've heard all sorts of things about mothers taking gin and nutmeg and the like but I wouldn't know how an abortionist performs an illegal abortion. They rupture the membranes somehow, I presume. Do it with a knitting needle or a button hook... The only time anyone

ever talked to us about it was a policeman. We had an
intruder in our garden one night and a policeman came up
and, blow me, we couldn't get rid of him! He started talking
about this particular woman that they knew of. We knew,
we knew her. Funnily enough, I'd had a delivery in her flat
with her daughter... But we kept quiet.

She was the only one – but she carried on because, you
know, later on, she was had up, wasn't she. She and her son
were had up for giving a woman a 'noxious substance to
produce an abortion'. What the noxious substance was,
though, I don't know.

Elizabeth C., who worked as a district midwife in Battersea, south
London, also described keeping her distance in order to protect
the abortionist from prosecution. Midwives often insinuated a
double message: the abortionist was creating life-threatening
disasters but she was also providing an important service for
women who were desperate not to bring another baby into an
already impoverished home:

Women did try to get rid of their babies while they were
pregnant. Oh yes, that happened a lot. They had brought
on a miscarriage or had one brought on and then they sent
for you and they thought it would be cleared, but often it
wasn't. It was awful.

I hated delivering a baby when it wasn't wanted. Ah, well
– after they were born they were often wanted... There was
one, she had her baby in the bucket. I wasn't going to tell
you but, you see, she was just going to have the baby and
let it drown. But she did accept it. It was the thought of
having them, I think. She was a bit simple.

They took castor oil to bring on a miscarriage, or hot gin,
I think, though I've forgotten actually. They could go to
somebody, a local woman, and pay and then we cleaned
up the mess, you see. But you never nursed them at home.
You sent them to hospital. You had to send them in
because they were liable to infection and lower pain. I
never knew exactly who was doing it. You didn't enquire
too far because they would have got prosecuted.

Elizabeth C.'s story of the woman trying to drown the baby brings
up the issue of infanticide. While infanticide did occur, we have
few references to it. Perhaps some of the accounts of premature
babies born in the toilet and babies accidentally smothered in bed

were not as innocent as they seemed. Handywomen were often said to have 'graveyard luck'. In other words, they were skilled at saving the mother but losing the child.[8]

Elizabeth C. also talked about women trying to leave their babies behind at the hospital:

> In hospital, you had to make sure they took their babies with them when they went out. They'd leave the baby behind. They didn't disown their babies so much at home as they did in hospital. Sometimes it would happen that they didn't want to take their babies home with them. Perhaps they were unmarried mothers, or...unhappy about having a baby. Maybe they had too many already at home. I don't know what it was, but you had to watch them.

The idea of purposely 'losing' or even killing one's baby may be shocking, but it is important to understand it within the context of women's lives in pre-NHS days when there was little or no contraception available to women. Yet another baby – if it survived – could bring even more poverty and ill-health to the woman. Working-class women were unlikely to allow themselves the luxury of sentimentality regarding pregnancy and babies, and abortion was an acknowledged but unspoken part of everyday life. While midwives were careful to distance themselves from abortion, they were well aware that both abortion and repeated pregnancies could have disastrous consequences for women's lives.

References

1. *Nursing Notes*, January 1928.
2. Cited in Kenner, Charmian, *No Time For Women*, Pandora Press, London, 1985, p.42.
3. Cited in Oakley, Ann, *The Captured Womb*, Basil Blackwell, Oxford, 1984, p.91.
4. Little, Bob, *Go Seek Mrs. Dawson – She'll Know What to Do*, unpublished thesis, University of Sussex, 1983.
5. Chamberlain, Mary, *Old Wives' Tales*, Virago Press, London, 1981.
6. Cited in *ibid*, p.120.
7. Untaped conversation with Elsie and Arthur Hunter, 1983.
8. Chamberlain, Mary, 'Life and Death', *Oral History – the Journal of the Oral History Society*, vol 11, no. 1, Spring 1983.

7 Unmarried mothers

> There was a terrible, terrible prejudice about all that kind
> of thing. A terrible stigma, and why I can't think because
> it takes two to make a bargain! It's always women who get
> the bad name.

In the first half of this century, an unmarried woman with a child
was seen as a disgrace to her family and a blot on the family name.
There was often strong pressure on the woman to conceal the
pregnancy from the eyes of the outside world, and bringing up
a child outside of wedlock could mean social isolation. However,
unmarried women had few options. Abortion was illegal and
dangerous. Adoption was complicated and expensive to arrange.

Often, the family coped by sending their daughter away to
relatives or to a 'mother and baby' home. At a safe distance from
the family neighbourhood, the baby could be placed in an
orphanage or offered for adoption. Often, though, the baby
would be integrated into the family with the grandmother acting
as mother. Since all women tended to hide their pregnancies
under loose clothing, in some circumstances it was possible for
the grandmother to appear to produce a 'late addition' to her
family. Bronwen, a Welsh midwife, remembers one such case:

> It was in 1926 during the two and a half years when I
> worked on the district. I have to laugh at these things.
> [giggles] I was visiting one of my mothers who had just had
> a baby when another lady came in – 'Ooh Nurse, will you
> come please? Grace is having an awful tummy-ache'.
>
> So I said, 'Yes, all right, I'll call. But wouldn't it be better
> to send for the doctor?' 'No', she said, 'you call and see her'.
> So after I'd finished with mother – this is in a terrace, of
> course – I went down to the first house of the terrace, and

there was Grace on a couch, an old-fashioned couch, having dreadful pains. You know, I'd seen dirty places before but I'd never seen one quite so dirty. It was dreadful, with frying pans and shoes under the table and a funny old stove, and the girl – she's a girl of about 17 – there on the couch.

I said to Mrs M., her mother, 'Will you go and fetch so-and-so for me?' And while she left the house I said to Grace, 'You know what's the matter with you, don't you?' She sort of said... 'No?' I said, 'Well, you're having a baby...' She nearly had a fit! Now, you see, boats used to come into the Swansea docks from foreign places. So she'd been out with one of the sailors and this was the baby.

I said 'Your mother will have to be told you know'. So Mrs M. came in and I said, 'You know what's the matter with Grace, don't you?' 'No', she says, 'no, I don't'. 'Well', I said, 'she's having a baby'. God, I think she would have killed her! So anyway, I calmed her down. I said, 'Now look, the baby's coming so just calm down, make yourself a cup of tea, and get plenty of water boiling'.

So anyway, after about two or three hours – I had thought I might have to send for the doctor, but anyway – the baby came and everything was all right. 'Now', I said, 'I want clean clothes, clean bed clothes, clean...' She said, 'I've got nothing for the baby'. I said, 'Well, that doesn't matter. Get me a nice clean sheet and a hot water bottle, not too hot'. So I did the baby up and wrapped it – lovely baby. And then I saw to the mother and I said, 'Now I want clean sheets to put on this couch...' The things we had to do, you know, it was dreadful. I attended her for about ten to twelve days. She got on quite well and the baby got on lovely.

Then about two years afterwards, I was in a council meeting and I looked round and there was Mrs M. with a bundle in her arms. I looked at her... 'Yes', she said, 'This is Mary! This is Grace's daughter!' And she loved that baby funnily enough. She took over looking after the child. The girl's mother took to the baby straight away. It was amazing, really. And she brought the child up. Anyway, she didn't murder her...like she threatened to!

Statistics for illegitimate births in the first half of the 20th century show a fluctuating pattern:

Illegitimate births in England and Wales for
women aged 15–44 years:

    1911–1920:   8.1   per 1,000 births
    1921–1930:   6.3   per 1,000 births
    1931–1940:   5.6   per 1,000 births
    1941–1950: 11.6   per 1,000 births[1]

These statistics do not show us how many women became
pregnant before marriage. Many of them would have procured an
abortion, had a hasty wedding or perhaps even committed suicide.
Elizabeth Roberts, in her oral history of working-class women in
north-west England, was told of several reported cases of pregnant
young women committing suicide by drowning.[2]

The women we interviewed made no mention of any personal
experience of pre-marital sex. It was always something that
happened to someone else and was often an awkward topic in
discussion. None of them had an illegitimate baby themselves, but
Ivy D. had two daughters, both of whom became pregnant in their
teens:

> Both my daughters got pregnant at 16 and that was terrible
> for me. I had to hide it both times. The first time would have
> been in the 1940s and the next time wouldn't have been
> till the 1960s 'cause I had J. very late in life. Both times it
> was all covered up. It was very shameful.
>
> When E. got pregnant, the first one, I was too scared to
> tell my husband at first. I lost weight with worrying about
> it. I couldn't tell anyone. When I did tell him, he was
> furious...with *me* really – for letting her go out so much. So
> he said, 'I'm going to lock her in the bedroom so that she
> can't go out.' But she climbed out of the window, over the
> roofs and out! [laughs] He'd previously done out her room,
> all in green, and he went up there and tore the curtains out
> and threw them out of the window. I never saw them
> again. Beautiful curtains, they were, so someone must have
> said, 'Thank you very much!'
>
> He kept locking her up but he didn't do it unkindly. He
> did it *for* her. I put her in a nursing home for unmarried
> mothers up at Blackheath, but then they 'phoned and said
> she'd run away. She wouldn't go back. She didn't like it
> there.

She had the baby in hospital and when she brought it home, my husband said, 'Don't make a fuss of it or she'll go and get pregnant again'. So I did what I was told and didn't hardly hold the baby in case she did. It was so upsetting. When my aunt came at Christmas we had to make out it wasn't ours. She said, 'Ooh, you've got a little baby!' I said, 'Yes, I'm just minding it'. She said, 'But it knows you a lot, doesn't it, Ivy'. [laughs] They all got to know after a while but they really looked down on E., like they did in those days. She never talks about it.

With my second daughter, we thought things would be different. You see, we were a bit better off. I'd saved some money from the little shops I ran, so I decided to get her educated. I thought, 'We'll have one that talks nice', so I never ever thought that she'd get pregnant! When she told me, all the blood ran from my face. I thought to myself, 'I can't tell my husband. He was so cross last time'. I never did tell him until after the baby was a month old. I paid for her to go into a home. I said, 'You'll have to have it adopted'. But she wrote to me from the home and said, 'Mum, they have to be perfect to be adopted, and he's got crooked toes, so I'll have to keep him'. [laughter] She really wanted to keep him – and I did too, really.

When I eventually told my husband, he pretended he knew. He didn't really. He thought she was staying with her sister. I warned my daughter, 'I'm telling dad today, so make sure T. [the baby's father] makes himself scarce 'cause I'm sure he's going to shoot him'.

Both times, I had no-one I could turn to, no-one I could talk to about it. It was terrible for me.

Support

Between the two world wars there were a number of voluntary organisations that worked with unmarried women and their babies. Some tried to place 'first offenders' in domestic service. In the mid-1920s, Lily O'Connell, a nurse, had an adoption arranged by the National Vigilance Association, an organisation that put single pregnant women in touch with adoption charities. It cost her £50, which she had to pay back to the Roman Catholic Church Orphanage over a number of years at 10 shillings a month.[3]

Adoption did not have legal status until 1926. Before then, it was arranged informally, often via local newspapers. The natural mother would advertise the child, and actually *pay* the adoptive parents either a weekly or a lump sum.[4]

Florence W., who worked as a midwife with the Salvation Army, recalls how women made varying decisions:

> Some of them were adopted and some of them kept the babies. There's all different kinds of people's circumstances. Some people come from very good circumstances and they have to go as far away as possible so that none of the neighbours or friends know about them. Sometimes these girls would change their minds and not have the babies adopted. There was a woman of 40 having her first child. She came right up to the last day when she was to have passed this baby over for adoption and then she couldn't go through with it. So then she told her story of how she was the subject of a bigamous marriage. So she decided against all the odds, against the relatives, to keep this boy. And that's what she did.

From their rhetoric, it was clear that the voluntary organisations felt it their duty to reform offenders and induce in them a sense of shame for their past behaviour. A woman who went to a church army home in 1918 gives an indication of the miserable circumstances there:

> Every day there we were marched through the streets for everybody to gaze at us and know we were single women expecting babies. It was terrible being stared at, with everyone knowing my shame. When we got back they put us to housework: washing up, cooking, cleaning, ironing and scrubbing. I was often hungry – they said we didn't need any extra food though we were carrying babies.[5]

An unmarried woman who did not go into a voluntary organisation home and who had no family support would often be forced to enter a workhouse to give birth. Florence W. has clear memories of such a case from her childhood in Great Yarmouth in the 1910s:

> The neighbour's daughter had twins and she wasn't married so she had to go to the workhouse. This is what happened then, you see. You had to go to the workhouse and that must have been terrible. And I can remember her now

bringing these twins home and sitting outside the house and everybody admiring them. She was received back into the family.

Bronwen H., who was married to a G.P. and practised as a midwife in Wales, remembers being called out with her husband to attend an unmarried young woman who did not quite make it to the workhouse when in labour:

> About 12 o'clock at night, the front door bell went and my husband answered it. 'Please, doctor, will you come at once'. So he said, 'Where is she?' The person said, 'She's in the Bridge Inn. I was taking her up to the workhouse to have this baby and she started having such pains. So she's in the Bridge Inn'. My husband said, 'You'd better come with me'. So just as well, off we went.
>
> The poor thing was in 'the snug' – a little room where someone who didn't want to see who was in the big room would take a jug and a pint of beer. You see, they'd put her in the snug. Well, my husband was quite a big man, tall man. He couldn't get through. She, poor dear, had struggled until you could only open the door about that much...so I had to make myself small and get inside...
>
> And the baby came... And I had to hang on to her tummy for a bit and my husband had to hand me the things though the door for me to tie the cord. The wife of the pub man brought me a nice soft towel and I managed to wrap the baby in this thing and put it on a hot water bottle while I saw to the mother. She was about 17 or 18. Anyway, I managed to open the door and handed out the baby. So she, bless her, was able to stand up, just about. And they were all put in a taxi and taken up to Surrey Lodge [the workhouse]. I don't know what happened to her and the baby after that.

After 1927, the Poor Law authorities had new powers that entitled them to detain those young unmarried women who were in receipt of poor relief when their child was born and classified as 'mentally defective'. In practice, this meant that many young women were locked away for life.

In psychiatric hospitals, it is not uncommon to meet women who, in the early part of the century, were locked away for no reason other than the fact that they had illegitimate children. Billie, one of the authors of this book, remembers:

During my nursing training I had to spend a month working in what was then known as a 'hospital for the mentally handicapped'. It was a huge institution in the north of England, miles from anywhere, almost like a village in its own right. On the geriatric ward were two old ladies who had been there since its days as a workhouse. They had been detained because they were unmarried mothers who were considered 'mentally subnormal'. The other situation I came across was in a psychiatric hospital, again an institution that had once been a workhouse. On the long-stay, psycho-geriatric ward was a woman who had been committed as insane during the 1910s. The only proof of her insanity was the fact that she had an 'illegitimate' child. According to her notes, there was no other evidence of mental health problems. She had just been conveniently shut away to protect her family's name. We were all told about her situation, but the doctors and nurses felt that she was now so affected by her 60-year long stay that she would be unable to cope with life outside, and so there she stayed.

The state might have had a single, inflexible approach, but the midwives we interviewed varied in their attitudes towards unmarried mothers. Some were reluctant to discuss the issue at all – no doubt a reflection of the denial and cover-up that existed around illegitimacy throughout their working lives. Nellie H., for example, a middle-class woman who was a midwife in private nursing homes, obviously found the subject distasteful and claimed that she had never come across an unmarried mother. At the other end of the scale, Florence W. devoted much of her midwifery career to working with single women in Salvation Army homes. There, midwives tried to educate the 'unfortunate women' and introduce them to a world of middle-class values and skills that would have been of debatable use to them:

> I've worked in those homes in all the big cities and it was very good work because you can help these people. Some of them are not trained how to even set a table when they come to you, so they got this training – housewifery and laundry, care of the baby and all that, which is invaluable for young girls who had never had any experience of that kind of thing.

Most of the midwives implied that working with unmarried mothers was something that cropped up throughout their working lives – a sad but inevitable part of life but not something to dwell on or discuss, something that was best 'swept under the carpet'.

Ninety-five year old handywoman, Mrs G., on the other hand, had no such qualms. She saw pregnancy as the price you paid for immoral sexual activity:

> Well, if they've had the sweets then they must have the sours, mustn't they?! Can't have yer sweets all of the time. They had to have their bottoms smacked, didn't they? Mind you, I wouldn't have liked to have had my bottom smacked when I was young!
>
> They had to go into homes, didn't they, and take their babies with them. Then when the babies grew up a bit, they had to go straight out to service. They had to go out and leave someone else to look after the baby.
>
> Mind you, there wasn't so many unwanted babies in them days – not like it is today.

Mother and baby homes

Several of the midwives we interviewed had worked in homes for unmarried mothers and their babies. From their accounts, it was clear that the homes varied greatly in the quality of care and help that they offered. Florence W. was very proud of the work carried out in the Salvation Army homes:

> They actually had their babies in the Salvation Army homes. They used to come two to three months before the child was born and stay three to four months afterwards. So you did their antenatal care, a doctor would come and see them, then the delivery, then the lying-in, and then the training of the girl to look after her baby afterwards. So we got to know them very well.
>
> At Bradwych, during the war, a lot of girls kept their babies and went into service and they used to keep in touch with the home. We used to call them 'associates'. And they used to come to a special function every year with the babies, some of them with quite older children. We kept in touch with them by correspondence and often got jobs for them. We did a lot of aftercare in those early days and your really felt as if you'd done something worthwhile.
>
> It was a house that belonged to some titled ladies and they made it into a maternity home, but we did have beds for three private patients, mainly farmers' wives that used to

come in from around there, and that was a nice little side-
line. They helped to finance the place. The girls didn't
have much money. We didn't have to employ any domestic
help because everybody did something. Some of them
would be there for six months. You didn't bar them 'cause
they couldn't pay. On the whole, they got on well together
'cause they had to share dormitories and I think some
made lasting friendships. But for some it was better to
make a fresh start without keeping in touch.

Midwives Josephine M. and Edith B. were not so impressed with
the work carried out in mother and baby homes:

Well, the City of London had a home for mothers and
babies at Stamford Hill and they worked them to death, they
really did. They had them about the City of London
cleaning and scrubbing – they kept them working right up
to the last minute of their pregnancies. Oh yes, and some
of these old home Sisters, they were right old battle-axes,
you know. 'You've got yourself pregnant but you're going
to pay for it while you're here.' And after that they got sent
back to the home and I s'pose the babies used to get
adopted. (*Josephine M.*)
    The first part of my midwifery training (in 1920, in
Newcastle) was with unmarried mothers and they were
very unkind to them. There was a terrible, terrible, prejudice
about all that kind of thing. A terrible stigma, and why I
can't think because it takes two to make a bargain! It's
always women who get the bad name. Of course, the
stigma very often left its mark on the child. I do remember
that the mothers were not allowed anything to ease their
pain, and if they had stitches – well, they just had stitches.
I think they'd have done forceps without an anaesthetic.
Usually, they were done under general anaesthetic – it was
ordinary chloroform or ether then. (*Edith B.*)

Family reactions

The families' reactions to unmarried mothers varied. Some families
seemed to be little affected, while others felt ashamed and angry.
Some eventually accepted the baby, but in other families the
feeling of disgrace was so great that the young woman and her
child were ostracised forever. Making a generalisation based on

our research, it would seem that working-class households were most able to accept illegitimacy. Edie M. explains:

> Amongst poor people like us I think more mothers would help their children if they got pregnant, rather than putting them away in a home. Yes, a case is coming to mind – Mary M., her name was. She got pregnant and the boy went to France for the '14–'18 war. And she had this little boy and the whole street stood by that girl.

Mary W. was a midwife in the pit villages around Barnsley, West Yorkshire, and she recalls:

> We did have unmarried mothers. Not a large proportion, but we did have them. The trouble with unmarried mothers was that very often they tried to conceal the pregnancy and a few times I've been called to the labour at the last minute without any warning during the pregnancy... I remember being called out to a girl who had worked all day and came home and had the baby that night.
>
> The babies were just sort of absorbed into the family. Not much stigma attached, no. The grandmother became the mother in most cases, and they were absorbed into the family. It didn't make much difference. The grandmother would look after the baby and the girl would go back to work – in the mills or domestic work. Very often there was a quick wedding so that the baby was legitimate.

Elsie B., a midwife from rural Devon, describes a situation familiar to all midwives. Throughout the centuries, midwives have had to cope with the contradiction of caring for people who lose wanted babies alongside supporting those who give birth to unwanted babies:

> I did have one that was sad, not from the unmarried mother's point of view, but from the next patient's point of view. The mother of the unmarried mother was standing there and all she kept saying was she hoped the baby would be born dead, but if it was born alive she hoped it would be all right. Of course, she was so upset about this. Anyway, needless to say, the girl had a good labour and a perfectly healthy baby. And the very next night we was called out to another person. That was a first baby, been married seven years and, needless to say, we had a stillborn

baby. No fault of anybody's you know, just one of these things that happened.

I remember one – I think the mother knew a few things. We were unlucky – it was a cord prolapse and of course we had a stillborn because mother had been pulling on the cord and she hadn't sent for anybody. I wondered about that.

As in today's society, sometimes the family itself could be a dangerous place for young women. Two of the midwives we talked to cited cases where women were pregnant due to incest. Josephine M. describes her horror of learning about such situations:

And that's another thing with these awful old men! Sometimes I remember women would be in having babies, perhaps they already had four or more children, and they would be desperate to get home. I remember this one woman. We tried to keep her in (perhaps she was a bit run-down or something) and she wouldn't stay. It appears – and apparently it's going on today, too – they couldn't leave their daughters at home with the old man. That was the first case I heard of. Of course, I was very green, only 21 years old. I didn't know anything of the outside world, being brought up in a close family in Ireland – but that did open my eyes. Oh yes, that sort of thing went on a fair old lot.

Florence W. also mentioned a case of incest:

When I was in Liverpool, we had a girl of 13 and her father was in jail because he was the father of her child... And she came from some little place in the heart of Wales. She had this baby that was perfectly normal and quite a big child, but although the mother was developed physically she wasn't developed mentally. So she was like a child and this baby was like a doll. But you can't get a baby like that adopted because of the incest – people worry that the child might have something wrong with it due to in-breeding. She was not allowed to go home because there were brothers...it was all most unsatisfactory.

She was in the care of the Salvation Army until she was 18, and the Children's Department helped to finance her. But she didn't seem to worry about it. She didn't seem a bit bothered that she was in this state. And none of the family ever came to see her. Eventually, they got her a little job in one of our Eventide homes there. But she wasn't much of a worker. Didn't have the brains to be educated.

Eventually, this baby went to Barnardos and I took it down from Liverpool on the train to Barnardos in Essex. And I often wondered what happened to that child.

During the Second World War, illegitimacy rates soared. Attitudes towards pre-marital and extra-marital sex relaxed and 'war babies' were more easily accepted, according to Katherine L. and Margaret A., midwives who worked near a US Army base in East Anglia:

There were a lot of unmarried girls here during the war. There were many American bases nearby and so they went out with the GIs. The illegitimate rate was very high but there was no stigma. It was accepted and they were absorbed into the family.

References

1. Cited in Lewis, Jane, *Women in England 1870–1950*, Wheatsheaf Books, Sussex, 1984, p.5.
2. Roberts, Elizabeth, *A Woman's Place – an Oral History of Working-class Women: 1890–1940*, Basil Blackwell, Oxford, 1984, p.76.
3. Lewis, Jane, *Women in England 1870–1950*, Wheatsheaf Books, Sussex, 1984, p.65.
4. *ibid*, p.64.
5. Humphries, Steve, 'Sex in a Cold Climate', *The Independent on Sunday*, 6 April 1991, p.27.

8 Wartime midwifery: 'everybody was for everybody else'

> ...a lot of the men were away and we liked to think we were holding the fort for them, looking after their wives.

In both world wars, women and children were the targets of governmental paternalism when the men went to the front. Ken W. remembers his mother, a handywoman, talking about the financial implications this had for her during the First World War:

> When the First World War broke out, my father volunteered like they all did, and she did tell me that she was never so well off as then. She got, I think, 18 shillings a week. She had six children under ten years old, and they gave a children's allowance. She told me that before the war he couldn't get work. So when the war came, he joined up as much for financial reasons as for patriotic reasons! Yarmouth was bombed by Zeppelins; one of the few places actually bombed in the First World War. I wasn't even born then...

In the Second World War, civilians were far more affected by air raids. In fact, until D-Day in 1944, more British civilians than soldiers died. The government took action to counteract the effect of war on the home front. One such action – evacuation programmes – highlighted the appalling state of health of women and children from inner-city areas. With men away at war and women employed to fill their jobs, the state could no longer expect 'the family', and women in particular, to take responsibility for the health and social needs of the community.

A new system of benefits came into effect, and the government passed bills to ensure a more even distribution of both money and food throughout the civilian population. The ensuing general improvement in health was reflected dramatically in both infant and maternal mortality figures.

Women who attended antenatal clinics were given certificates that entitled them to an extra half ration of food, and mother and child welfare centres sold various items at subsidised prices:

> We could buy things cheap from the clinics – orange juice, virol, Bemax [wheatgerm], that sort of thing. You only paid about fourpence for a bottle of pure orange juice. I went to the clinics for these things, but not to go by all the things that they told you you should be doing. I think a mother should learn to use her own initiative myself. (*Lou N.*)

Evacuation

At the beginning of the Second World War, the government made hasty plans to evacuate all pregnant women and their children from the cities and large towns to the comparative safety of rural areas. In fact, less than one-tenth of the women who were expected to take up the scheme responded, and almost all of those who did returned home as soon as they were able. Alice F. remembers having pressure put upon her to be evacuated:

> Oh, they kept on and on, right. The town hall kept coming down to me. He said, 'I think that you should go away 'cause you're the only person down here with a child'. I said, 'I know, but I still have a mother and father that I worry about'. So he said, 'I can understand, but we're thinking of the baby'. I said, 'Naturally, you're thinking of the next generation to take over'. I said, 'Another war, you know...'

Midwife Edie B., who worked for 50 years in a maternity home in West Norwood, south London, describes urban women's dislike of being forced to live in the country:

> In 1940, we were bombed so we moved to Tring – Lord Rothschild's place, very posh. There used to be all these bombs flying about London, so we used to take the mothers out there to have their babies. Every week they used to bring a carload of expectant mothers up, you see. But when the mothers had had their babies and they were allowed out again, they were longing to get back to London – in all the turmoil! They used to say, 'We cannot stand this 'orrible

'ush! Somebody rattle a tin can or something!' Homing instinct. They couldn't stand the country.

We had a woman come in, and she'd been in a raid, and she'd had an arm blown off three or four weeks previously. And she came in and had a perfectly normal baby. It never interfered with her pregnancy. They used to come in, frightened to death, but then they wanted to go back home.

Florence W., working in the Salvation Army has similar memories of womens' dislike of evacuation:

During the war we had an evacuation centre out of London. We went to Bragborough, near Rugby, right out in the heart of the country, and that was supposed to be used for part two midwifery training, you know, straightforward cases. And then we had Willesley Castle in Matlock. The Mothers' Hospital took that over for several years. These people used to come up in a coach and stay in billets in the village, then come up to the big house for antenatal care and deliveries. But nearly all of them, when they delivered, went back home. These women who were sent for evacuation, if they were Londoners, they didn't like it. They didn't want to stay in the villges. They wanted to get back home. They didn't have any bingo, any fish and chip shops, any cinema. And it was all arranged so hurriedly.

On the whole, midwives seemed to like working in the evacuation centres, where they were the sole practitioners in charge of normal births. For Esther S., a working-class midwife who had spent her life in the city, evacuation opened up a wealth of new experiences:

When I moved to Portsmouth to finish my training, we were all in a high explosives area. A lot of the mums were evacuated out to the country, and I went out with them, to Liphook. Liphook's lovely. We went to a big country house there; it was beautiful. And we had what we thought would be the 'normal', not 'at risk' (abnormal) mums. Normal and abnormal – it sounds awful, doesn't it, to speak like that. They used to say that in those days. They don't so much now. It's 'at risk' and 'not at risk', isn't it? So we used to have those that we felt would be straight-forward. Occasionally, we had to have a doctor out. I have known them with a retained placenta brought back into St.

Mary's (hospital) but normally the majority of them just delivered and all was well.

It was lovely. I loved it out there. It was a big country house, a different way of living. You saw the idea of nature around you as well. The lovely trees... Oh, it was gorgeous... Magnolia trees...and we had lovely country walks round there. And we were very friendly, us girls, with the two postwomen in the war with the men gone, and we were waiting for our letters and that...and they'd come out on a Sunday for those that were off duty and take us for walks. They knew all the country walks. They were lovely girls. We did like them. They were two sisters and they became the postmistresses. So I liked the evacuation days.

Midwife Nellie H., who worked mostly in private maternity homes, paints a different picture. She describes the disruption that evacuation could cause, as well as the spirit of co-operation in the face of hardship that it could also engender:

Dr K. asked me if I'd like to go with the women to somewhere in the Midlands. So I said, 'Oh all right', I would try it and I would come back if I didn't like it. In those days, when you were evacuated during the war, you didn't know where you were going. All the names and signposts had been taken down from everywhere and you had no directions where to go. Only the driver knew where he was going, but even he didn't know the district, so it was a terrible business. We went up there, this was in 1940. And the driver said, 'I don't know where I'm going to take you. I've got a name here, but I don't know it, and I've never heard of it'. So, I had one nurse and meself in there with about 48 pregnant women. And the nurse had been up all night, she told me. So I said, 'Well, dear, you'd better lay down and go to sleep. There's no reason for you to stay awake'.

Well, we got part of the way up there and one of the girls started in labour! I could see what was happening, you see, so I said to the driver, 'If you see a hospital anywhere near, take her in, because we don't want a baby born in the coach'. It would have been a bit of a business, wouldn't it? Can you imagine...up there with all the other mothers around!

So he stopped at a hospital on the way, but I couldn't tell you which hospital because there was no names anywhere.

And they took her in and kept her there and apparently she
had the baby in about a couple of hours. So it would have
been born on the way! And I didn't want a baby born. I
mean, I didn't mind, but I mean, it would have been a bit
embarrassing for the driver – and all the mothers. Might
have frightened the life out of them, mightn't it – if it was
their first baby!

We went to a little village near Leicester, it was, and I was
there for about a fortnight. The matron there had previously
been in charge of a district up there and she wasn't used to
ration cards or anything like that and she was a bit lost. She
didn't know quite what to do, so I think I was a great help
to her because I'd been used to ration cards on the district
before I went up there. She said, 'Oh, I am glad you came,
Miss H., because I don't know anything about it. But there
was nobody else that would take the job on'. It was only a
small home. They were going to have about twelve mothers
and babies. It was a little country house that somebody had
given up. They'd gone away and left it for us.

When I'd been there about a fortnight – I was running
around with bedpans – the Medical Office of Health came
and asked me to go and run a small maternity unit so I went
and I was there for five years. It was part of a big estate that
belonged to the C. family. The man, Mr C., was gone to the
war, and his mother still lived there and they turned part
of it into a hospital for mothers. That's what I mean,
people were ever so good. In the war, everyone was
marvellous. You never heard of anyone who wouldn't give
you a helping hand. Really marvellous, they were. And the
people of London, especially the East Enders, they were
marvellous people. They used to come up and stay a
fortnight. We used to try and get them billeted afterwards
at Lockington or Derby, or somewhere near there, but
they'd say, 'No, we've got to go home. We might be wanted
there'. So they went home with their new babies!

Air raids

Women's memories of the Second World War often revolve
around air raids. Here, Alice F. describes conditions during air raids
in London and the effect on her and her new baby:

When the war came and there were air raids, you'd have
to grab your baby and run. It happened one morning with

the baby in the bath, and I had to grab him, throw a towel round him, and run up the garden and get in that shelter. And of course, I'm worried sick, and I'm thinking, 'Oh, this baby, will he catch a cold', you know...but it was a good thing that we did get in there because they bombed us two doors away and they were all killed. We were lucky that we had this shelter built right down into the earth – and I bought a bed, proper bed, mattress to go on it and I fixed his little bed up in the corner, and me dog come down with me...and I think that saved us...

It had a steel gate on the door. And when the fireman called in, 'Are you all right in there, 31?' 'Yes, quite all right.' 'Don't come out, there's a time bomb in your garden.' I thought, 'Oh!... What?' He come back and he said, 'The time bomb is...an alarm clock! But you've got no street doors and no windows, all blown off up the main road. And I think your street door's completely blown off. Boom!' Yes, nobody knows what that war was.

I met a young girl. It had just stripped her of everything that she stood in. I took her indoors and I wrapped her up in a blanket. And I said, 'You'd better stay with us, love'. And I said to my friend, 'Oh, what a life, but I am worried about my little Malcolm'. So she said, 'Don't worry, I think he's a strong baby'. But it was all that sort of thing that used to worry me. And I used to try to do my bathing at a different time, but this blasted Hitler! He bombed us all of one day, 24 hours, non-stop. You couldn't go out, you couldn't do anything. It was frightening.

We used to have a big sort of case to put your baby in. What they'd given these things to us for was because they always thought we were going to be attacked by gas. This was to stop the baby breathing it in like those poor souls over there in Russia [Chernobyl] at the moment. That's what would have stopped them and that's why we had the gas masks, too. You had to pump it to keep the air going to the baby. *BUT*, the point is – which I don't think the government had thought of – if the mother, or whoever had got that baby, left off pumping, it would die! Now what was the point of that! S'pose the mother got hit, where was the baby?

Of course, *my* baby christened it!! [laughing] When my mother saw it, she said, 'Oh dear, has he got to go in there?' So I said, 'Get him in'. And he loved it! Laughing away. And there was me at the side, pumping and pumping the thing. It was like a big box with a cover on, all fixed in, and you could see your baby, there was a lovely opening. Oh, he loved it, kicking away, wee-ed in it and all!

And I'll always remember it. My husband had come home at one time from France and he said, 'You haven't got one of these boxes?' And I said, 'Well, we're going to get one'. He says, 'Well, I'll pull the bloomin' town hall down if you don't get one!' And of course there was no end of mothers all lining up for one of these things when we heard what it was for, that the Germans had started using gas. Of course, naturally, the government gave them out. And of course we had to return them...and all the rest of it...

It used to be very funny because you'd get a policeman riding on a bike with a notice on his back – '*ALL CLEAR!*' Oh dear!

Midwives described their experiences of having to go out to home births during air raids in the blackout. Mary T. described for us with pride her friend Elsie Walkerdine's bravery in going out to births in Deptford during air raids:

Four foot ten inches, she was, but she coped with the biggest. One man came round one night during the war. He said, 'Nurse, as soon as the 'all clear' siren goes, come and see the wife. She is bad'. She said, 'I'll come along now, father. You 've come along for me, I'll come along for you'. And he had a saucepan over his head!

She went one night during a raid, and she said it seemed as though the plane was almost following her, gunning her. Nothing kept Nurse Walkerdine at home.

Changes brought by war

The war affected midwifery in many different ways, and its repercussions were felt by midwives for many years afterwards. One interesting change – in postnatal care of mothers – came about as an indirect result of the war experience. Margaret A. explains:

Back in the early '30s we'd keep 'em in bed for at least twelve days, then gradually it went down to ten days, but when I did my first refresher course, there were two sisters there from the Salvation Army hospital in Hackney – the Mothers' Hospital – and they told tales of getting their mothers out of bed after delivery as soon as the mothers felt like it, during the bombing in London. They'd been doing it all through the war. The mothers were allowed to get up, pick their babies up and *run*. And they'd had such success that they kept on with it! – 'early ambulation'. Well, as soon as I heard that, I came home here and I started 'early ambulation', without any reference to the doctors or anyone. Of course, it cut down on DVTs. [Deep vein thromboses are blood clots in the veins of the leg that can be caused by keeping women in bed after childbirth. DVTs can move throughout the bloodstream and block vital organs such as the lungs, causing death.]

Wartime spirit

Midwives and other women whom we interviewed waxed lyrical about the way in which people were brought together by the 'wartime spirit'. Midwife Esther S. remembers:

I think the thing about the babies and mums was the happy atmosphere about it all. I mean, the war to me was the happiest years of my life – terrible thing to say it, but it was. I mean, nobody had a grudge about anybody else. You were wonderful together. Everybody smiled…(and there was nothing to smile about sometimes) – but you knew that today you were here, tomorrow you were gone, and you couldn't afford to fall out with anybody because you never knew if we'd meet again. It was wonderful. Everybody would say, 'The war years were the happy years for the way that people lived'. No bickering, no nothing. I mean, they all got down into the shelters and the child was as important as the mother, I mean, nobody said, 'I was in 'ere first'. Everybody moved up a bit nearer for somebody else to push in. You know, everybody was for everybody else. Marvellous! I loved all that spirit in the war.

Mum in the war – she had a hard time really when she was pregnant. There was the awful worry of Dad being at war and they never knew when their letters were going to come – all those long silences. It was terrible. You were often in tears because somebody said, 'Have you heard the news? Well…we've heard a rumour…and …' It was terrible really, so you had to keep them up, you know, keep going with them. They were lovely people.

Many of the midwives we interviewed intimated that during the war they had taken on a new role of authority within the community; namely the one that was usually accorded to men. Mary W. explains:

> Then of couse there were a lot of men away and we liked to think we were holding the fort for them, you know, looking after their wives...

In a similar vein, Esther S. describes her wartime involvement with families:

> In the war you found that not only did you do your midwifery, you were their friend as well. You had to be. You had to be their moral support because the dads weren't there and sometimes if the families were all separated, they looked on you as the figure head almost. You'd do all sorts of things for them. And you know...talk with them. In fact, I found that visits got very long, but you didn't mind because there was no social life in the war really. Only dances if you could get together with the troops when they were in... But you see, you just made your life in your families and homes, because half the time you were in the shelters. We used to talk together about all sorts of things. They all listened to you, and they liked your ideas.

One of the recognised problems in recording oral history is that of selective memory. People tend to tell the stories they want to remember, and nowhere, it seems, is there such a vested interest in remembering the positive than when it comes to the topic of wartime. All the women we interviewed, including the midwives, tended to gloss over or omit the unsavoury aspects of living in a country that could, at the very least, be described as suffering from severe disruption.

It is important to place oral history in the context of its socio-political background and whilst women's positive memories of wartime may well be due in part to the coming together of people in the face of a common enemy, plus the aforementioned improve-ment in diet and living conditions, it is nevertheless worth remembering that war also brought with it a whole lot of factors that induced misery and despair. Books that we read about the period make it clear that illegitimacy, venereal disease, rape, prostitution, marriage and divorce rates all soared during both the

First and Second World Wars. We found that women did not want to be drawn into discussion about such things.

'My first delivery'

It seems fitting to end this chapter with Esther S.'s enthusiastic description of her first single-handed midwifery experience. The event took place during an air raid in the Second World War:

> I was getting to the end of my training in Croydon out on the district. I loved it, I really loved it. I was beginning to know midwifery a little bit – I don't think you ever do until you're a midwife out on your own...
>
> My midwife was called Mrs Treasure and I think she thought I had a little bit of sense. I don't know but she used to leave me a lot on my own, anyway. The biggest thrill of my life was when I knew I was going to do my first delivery on my own on the district.
>
> Of course, now it wouldn't be so bad, but it was the times we were living in. You didn't only have to cope with mum and baby, you had to cope with, well, everything. Keep yourself safe, so that you arrived – I mean, no good you pegging out on the way there, was it! You had to get there. You had to go through the middle of the night with all the flying bombs, on a bike with a cover over your headlamp. It was the blackout. And you wore navy blue, which I thought was dreadful because there were no lights anywhere. It was pitch black. You get a very dark night with no moon and there's nothing anywhere, absolutely pitch black!
>
> Well, this particular delivery of mine, which was really the highlight of my life, I'll never forget it. To me it was wonderful. Mrs T. sent me out one day and she said, 'Now, I'm not going to give you any work to do this morning. I'm going to do the work, but you've got to go round to three mothers that might deliver and you've got to get very familiar with how you find the roads in the night because, as you know, it'll be pitch black. Really get familiar with it. Find the house, knock on the door, see the mum and tell her that you'll be coming in the night should she want you, and they've got to 'phone you, and tell them all that they've got to do'.
>
> That took me a morning to do those three because I had to find them and get really familiar with the roads and

thinking, 'Now, if it's lightish, what will my landmarks be? If it's not light, how will I find it?' – you know, little tiny bits of paper with a little torch so I could just see! Write meself little notes – no one else to ask – usually there wasn't a soul about!

So that particular night I went to bed all apprehensive. Now, the bed was underneath a Morrison shelter, d'you know? A table shelter – they were sort of iron, you see, dark green and very strong. Down the side there was more metal and then a little bit of strong mesh for air, and then there was a hole where you got underneath and the back was all filled in and then more mesh at the other end. Well, you were supposed to lay two people lengthways in those, but of course where I was billeted out there was 'Mum', 'Dad', and Pam (lovely girl). They were doing an important job and didn't have to go to war, but her brother and sister had gone out. They were fighting. So there was four of us, you see, so what could we do? So we decided that as we had a great big huge table in that room as well, 'Dad' would get under that every night – though, what protection it would be I dunno! – and 'Mum', Pam and I got underneath the Morrison. But we couldn't lay lengthways because it wasn't big enough so we had to lay widthways – that meant to say our feet were out so we each took a two-hour stint of being awake to call the others when the raids come on and you all had to lift your legs in – 'cause we said it would be no good if you got your legs chopped off! Say it would be my stint, you had to sit up to keep awake for two hours. We did this in turn each night.

Well, this particular night when the 'phone went, I was asleep and Pam said, 'Nurse, the 'phone's ringing. I expect it's for you'. And when I answered the 'phone it was one of these three patients.

Well, I had to get all round the back of the house to get me bike out and lock it all up, get meself out, take a bag and that. And I had to ride alongside of the park and there was a warden and he said, 'Get off the bike. They're falling fast. Listen to them, all coming over!' I said, 'Can't. Maternity case...' And rode on ever so cocky! I went on and them doodle-bugs kept stopping. They're terrible, when they stop. They swish on down, you see, and then they fall, and of course they shatter roads – a road went like a pack of cards! The devastation! You'd hear them coming, the plane's noise, and then they stopped – swish – and when they stopped you had to do something because they'd drop anywhere. Many of a time I've been near them and you just laid down flat on the road, so I just fell off the bike, laid down – there's no traffic about but say there had been, they wouldn't have seen you on a dark night in the middle of the road – they'd have rolled over you...

Well, I got to this house finally because it was a shocking night, one of the worst they'd had. I got to this house and I moved along, fumbled me way along and found the door and put me bike in the gate, took me lamp off to check it was the right number and I knocked and nobody came. And I was ever so frightened. So I pushed the door and it was open so in I go and I fumbled around to try and find Mum and I couldn't find anybody! Suddenly Dad came in from the garden and he said, 'Oh good. I'm glad you've come, Nurse, we're all in the shelter. What a terrible night!' So he said, 'Come in'. So I get into the kitchen. And he said, 'We can't have any of her nice stuff. That's all upstairs and I'm too frightened to go up and get it'. I said, 'Oh, never mind, we'll have all the bowls and stuff from the kitchen. Don't worry to go upstairs, for goodness sake!' Because he'd got four children, four little girls.

Down the bottom of the shelter he'd made it that there were like two shelves and there were two little girls on one shelf and two on the other, one either end. Lovely little girls. Anyway, there was Mum lying on the bunk and there was another bunk entrance, so I just got in and looked at her, you see, and I said 'Well, I think what we'd better do is get everything to the shelter that we can think of. Then we won't have to go out. If the water's cold, it's just cold and that's it'. So he said, 'Well, before it got too bad I brought down that great big jug you put cold water in'. They hold eight pints, you know, the old jugs and basins on the old washstands. Marvellous, great boon. Well, they had one of those jugs, didn't have a basin. So I said, 'Well, fill that with water and I'll get down in this Anderson (you know, they were dug right down) and you pass everything down to me and I'll take it and then when you've finished you come on down. He said, 'There's an upturned bucket. You can sit on there for a seat'. So I sat on it – had a bit of a rim round me! He got ready to give me that water, and just as he was about to give it to me the doodle-bug had stopped and it was coming down – swishing – any minute it was going to drop. I mean, you didn't know where it's going to land. And so what did he do? He was so frightened he fell and he tipped eight pints of cold water over me! From head to foot, I was absolutely drenched! Right, of course, he cried, he was in such a state. Me dripping wet from head to foot. Well, what could I do, I just laughed! And it was all mud underneath, you see. It was earth and it just made it into all slosh!

The mother said, 'Well, you can't stay like that!' I said, 'No, well, I'll have to get some of these clothes off', because I was wringing wet. Well, we'd lost all the water and we've to go up to get more water, so she said, 'You'd better go up. In the kitchen there's my clothes that I dropped out of on the floor'. So I dressed in her maternity clothes in the kitchen! Didn't care whether Dad could see what I was doing or not! I undressed in the kitchen! He said, 'I won't look'. I said, 'You can't see if you did!' It was pitch black. He said, 'Where are you?' I said, 'I'm finding the clothes!' Oh! Nothing so funny in all of my life! So I go down in her maternity clothes! And he had to proceed to get some more water. I don't think I ever got any hot water from beginning to end.

Anyway, he'd made little curtains across the bunks and these little children kept looking out at me. And I said, 'Now look, if you're very good when the baby comes you can open the curtains when I tell you and have a look...'

We carried on, and Mum was delivered on the bunk, no stitches, and Dad was wonderful. He was in a terrible state about what he'd done to me. I said, 'Don't be silly – that's nothing!'

Anyway, she was marvellous and the baby was born and it was a boy and she'd told me that she was going to call it Richard if it was a boy. And I said, 'We've got Richard!' And I said, 'Children – you've got a little baby brother'. And d'you know, it was just like out of comic cuts. They all pulled the little curtains back – this is true! – they pulled the little curtains back and had a little look out!

And I said 'I'll bring the baby over and show you in a minute'. And they were awake all that time. And I took the baby over, pulled the curtains back, they had a look and then they went to sleep. We never heard another word.

About 4 o'clock in the morning, the doodle-bugs stopped because it was light. Dawn coming, they didn't come on over then.

Of course, it takes a long time to clear up when you're down in a place like that. Where d'you start? We got Mum over onto the clean bunk, did all this, that and the other.

That was my most wonderful delivery. All on my own. I mean, when you think of it, that wasn't bad was it?

Of course, my midwife had said, 'If you don't want me in the night for any reason, let me know about 8.30 a.m. and we'll sort out the work'. Well, by the time I'd finished everything there, I'd forgotten about my clothes. Elated I was! You won't believe this. I put on my coat – navy blue gabardine mac in those days – and a storm cap, on top of Mum's clothes, and left her and went on.

It was about seven in the morning when I finished and I thought, 'Oh, I must tell my midwife – had my first baby!' So I went by her door and I knocked. And she looked out of her bedroom window and she said, in her posh accent, 'What's the matter, Nurse?' And I said, 'Nothing. I've delivered a baby'. She said, 'Well, I don't want to know at 7 o'clock in the morning'. 'Oh, but it's lovely!' So she said, 'What *have* you got on?' She saw all these clothes hanging down! 'Oh', I said, 'I've got mother's maternity clothes on'. 'Course they were so big and they just dropped below my mac! She thought I was a nutcase, I think. Anyway, I had to go back at 8.30 a.m. and explain what had happened.

But, I mean, oh dear, oh dear, that was a wonderful delivery though. You can imagine can't you. I was absolutely elated!

9 Working lives: the effect on childbearing women

> I lost my babies through poverty – going to work. But there was nothing for it. You had to work.

Although many women did paid work in the period between the wars, much of it was casual or home-based, especially for working-class women. So it was not recorded in official statistics. Hence, the 1931 census stated that only 10 per cent of married women had paid work.[1]

Common jobs for women were taking in washing, ironing, mangling, cleaning and child minding. This type of work could be fitted in around a woman's home life, especially her own child care needs, and provided vital extra money. Lou N. remembers:

> When I first started work (at 14) I was a coil winder. Then I was a french polisher. Next I was a brush maker – yeah, that used to cut your fingers, that did, brush making. But, of course, once you got married and had kids you couldn't fit these jobs in so I had to go cleaning flats and offices. I was in one job for 22 years, cleaning Social Services.
>
> I worked even when the kids were little. It was the only way. I couldn't live on his money 'cause a barman was the worst-paid job out, it was.

Edie M. talked about a job to which she returned *with* her baby, who was only a few weeks old:

> He went onto the dole and I went and did washing for half a crown a day. I worked from about ten in the morning to four o'clock at night at Miller's Yard. They were the people that had neighbouring stalls next to us, Italian fruiterers, they were. I used to go and wash for them for half a crown a day. I used to take me baby in an old-fashioned wooden push-chair with a bit of carpet on the seat. I used to put the

132

pram in the doorway, put the copper in the corner of the room, light it, then start the washing. They had great big sheets, these Italians, luxurious beds, and she'd keep throwing more things out the window – 'Here y'are, Ede'. Later, I went and got a job at Millers in Gray's Inn Road, washing up and that, and then somebody minded the baby.

Domestic work was demanding and exhausting. The tasks were repetitive and tedious, with women having to stand for hours on end. Hard physical labour coupled with an inadequate diet had disastrous effects on women's health, and hence on their pregnancies and births. It is important to remember that the women we interviewed have all lived into their seventies, eighties and even nineties, but there were many other women who died early in life, often from the consequences of poverty.

Jane W. describes working throughout her pregnancy:

That was in 1925. I'd stayed at work till I was six months pregnant, working as a machinist down Tooley Street – Army & Navy Territorial Outfitters – a good firm to work for. And then, at that time – I don't know if you'll remember the Charleston garters that came out top fashion, all frills and bells and bows – well, my aunt, she had this little draper's shop and she asked me if I could make up these garters for her, so I used to do that. But really, perhaps I should have been resting more? I don't know. Anyway, I got over it.

It is not necessarily harmful to work during pregnancy. In fact, the reverse is often the case. However, the type of work undertaken by pregnant, working-class women – whether the hard physical slog of washing or the painstakingly delicate activity of doing needlework in a sweatshop – certainly was detrimental to their health.

There was no maternity leave, and many women had to return to demanding jobs soon after childbirth. Outside of the professions, terms and conditions of employment were poor or non-existent. Edie M. attributes the death of two of her babies to returning to work too quickly after the births:

My first baby was a beautiful baby, right up to ten months old when I lost her. Every time I took her on the bus, people said, 'Oh what a lovely baby!'

During that time we had extreme poverty. My husband was on the dole and we lived in one tiny little room without running water or sanitation. So I got a job in Whitechapel, washing up again. They had a big night trade there, and when I went in in the morning there'd be a great big wooden sink full of plates, piles and piles of plates, and I used to have to stand on a box to reach 'em.

I left the baby, and my husband being out of work, he used to mind her. Well, what happened was, it must have been 1921, we got an extreme summer then and [gastro]enteritis started. Any rate, she was taken to Bancroft Road Hospital and to cut a long story short, I lost her there. Fifty babies died in that ward that week from 'enteritis. So I lost my baby. They brought her round in this little white coffin beside the bed, and I bought some flowers and put them there and they told me I shouldn't have done it 'cause it turned her. When I went to look at her again she was discoloured under there. They said, 'You shouldn't have put flowers in the coffin'. I slept with that coffin a week there... People wouldn't realise it, would they?...

I think I had an empty brain as a teenager. But it wasn't empty when I lost my first baby. I walked the streets at night for about six weeks – missing her, missing holding her, missing washing the nappies, missing getting her ready before I went to work in the morning... It was a nightmare.

My third baby, Freddie, I lost him at 13 months, but he had wasting disease on and off. I was just pulling him out a bit, he was getting a nice, normal little boy, and then he developed pneumonia. He'd been ill all the time I had him so I suppose I recovered from that quicker than the first one. A sad little baby he was. One part I don't like to remember was when I went to see him when he was dying. That baby, he was so lovely...he was 13 months and knew me so well. My baby was dying...and he put his little arms out and tried to get to me as I sat beside the bed... That won't go, that memory...

So I lost the third one, too. But only through poverty, going to work. I think if I'd stayed at home I wouldn't have lost that first one because she wouldn't have been minded by her dad and developed gastroenteritis. And I wouldn't have lost the second one if I hadn't gone to work. They say if you breast-feed it gives them protection, but he went into the nursery at two weeks old. There was nothing else for it. You had to work unless – well, I s'pose you could stay at home and manage on bread and marg or something...

Edie had a creche place for some of her children. The creche was near where she worked, a kitchen in Drury Lane, and her employer contributed to its cost. At the time, creches were quite unusual. However, later on, in wartime, when the state wanted women's labour, nurseries and creches became readily available:

> I was working in Drury Lane at the time. The creche closed for holidays, so I used to put him in a little box beside me in the kitchen, and we used to keep putting his dummy into syrup or something. And that's how we got over the week or fortnight's holiday when the creche was shut. Our missus used to contribute to that creche. Got a place in it, nine pence a day. And I used to have to come right the way from Dulwich on a tuppenny tram to get the baby in. D'you know, I've stood waiting in Essex Road, holding my baby in a shawl, on a foggy morning, 7.30, to get up to the Kingsway by eight, get it in the creche. Sometimes I think to meself 'Oh poor babies'. It's wrong innit? Well, it *was* wrong. I never had the pleasure of bringing them up.

Although combining the roles of mother and worker was difficult, it would be wrong to paint a picture of all women resenting their working lives. For many women, work meant time away from the home, a sense of freedom and pride. Despite her gruelling experiences, Edie M. says:

> Me life was at work. All me fun was at work.

Women in the home

The overriding ideology of the period between the wars was very much that 'a woman's place is in the home'. Women's magazines of the period reinforced this attitude. The first issue of *Woman's Own* in 1932 described itself as 'Our new weekly for the modern young wife who loves her home'.[2] For middle-class women who had access to the new gadgets on the market, housework became a science. Women were encouraged to stay at home and create a cosy nest, adorned with hand-crocheted doilies and home-made cakes, from which their husbands and children could blossom forth into the world. Pregnant women were exhorted to take up embroidery to while away the hours:

> Surely there is no more delightful task than preparing an
> outfit for the Little Stranger. The wee garments are so
> dainty and easy to make, and as we stitch into them all the
> best wishes in the world, we wonder perhaps if we are
> working for some boy or girl who will one day become a
> national hero or heroine.[3]

As well as being the ideal homemaker, middle-class women faced
another pressure. They also had to be desirable at all times.
Magazines of the period contain many articles citing the dire consequences of 'letting yourself go':

> I will not listen to the little housewife who tells me that she
> is so busy looking after the house that she has no time to
> 'bother about herself'. That is sheer bunkum and a woman
> with that point of view deserves all the heartbreak that is
> coming to her.[4]

Such messages had very little meaning for most working-class
women. For them, working in the home was a never-ending
succession of grinding tasks – beating carpets, scrubbing floors,
blacking hearths, washing and mangling. The impossibility of
winning the battle against dirt meant that there was often an
emphasis on outside appearances. The step was always clean,
the doorknob was always polished and the girls had to have
clean pinafores. One midwife, Bronwen H., who worked in Wales,
remembers with awe, standards of cleanliness achieved against all
the odds:

> A woman with eight babies, and she was a tiny wizened little
> thing. But her place was absolutely spotless. Poor thing, I
> don't know how on earth she managed it...and the children
> were beautifully clean, very poor, of course, but the table
> and all that, beautifully clean. Another mother...she had
> about four or five children and she used to sweep all the
> floors and there was a hole in the wooden floor – and
> she'd just sweep everything down into the hole! How they
> survived, I don't know...I just don't know...

Feeding a family

In the 1920s and 1930s, most people did not possess refrigerators
so buying, preparing, preserving and storing food was a major part
of domestic work. Fresh food had to be bought daily, often
entailing a long walk to the cheapest shops or street market. It was

a time-consuming and tedious task, and all the more exhausting if several children were in tow and there was a heavy pram to push.

Poverty meant little choice in food, but the women we interviewed were proud of their ability to 'make do' and concoct something appetising to put on the table. Midwife Esther S. remembers:

> People lived ever so poor, but they didn't waste, that's the thing. They always managed to make a meal out of something. They did all sorts of things to make sure that there was always a meal on the table for their husbands to come home to. Even if it were two penn'orth of chidlings, they'd fry them up, p'raps put them on a piece of toast... Often the women themselves would go without...

Jane W. reinforced this idea:

> There were 14 of us kids. I never saw my mother have a dinner. We'd all sit round the table, and she'd be like a waitress, giving it all out, passing it on. Whether she had any before or after, I'll never know. I don't think she did when I look back. She worked really hard to feed us lot.

Edie M. remembers 'making do' with whatever food was available. She describes a period in her life when she shared this task with a neighbour:

> I always cooked a hot dinner. I can remember getting a pound of chops for sixpence so you could have them with potatoes and get a dinner for about ninepence. We didn't have meat every day. One of my famous dinners was three penn'orth of bacon bones, put on with lentils and we'd have a whacking fine pot of stew.
>
> When I lived in Clerkenwell – just one room with a table, two chairs, a bed and a gas stove – I had a neighbour downstairs, Mrs W. She had three boys and a girl. We used to take it in turns inviting each other up. I'd call down, 'Mrs W...' and she'd come up with the children and share my stew. Next day, she'd call up to me and we'd have a big plate of hers! [laughs]

Housing

Housework was doubly difficult because much of the housing stock was in a very poor condition. Mary W., a midwife, describes the conditions in a Yorkshire mining village:

Most people were in terraced housing. The council houses were only just starting to be built, so there was a lot of really old housing. No indoor sanitation. It was the exception rather than the rule if they had a bathroom. No indoor toilets – outside privies. Lighting was mainly gas, though we had parts of the village that had oil lamps. Of course, it was a colliery area so there was plenty of coal. The miners get an allowance of coal and so the houses were well heated. Very often, for the birth, they would bring the bed down into the living room and the woman would stay in bed (or at least she told me she stayed in bed; we had this strict rule at that time about a woman staying in bed for eight days) and she would supervise her domestic arrangements from the bed – and very well too. I should imagine, looking back, it did them good, too, because, for example, I once went in and the woman was kneading a stone of bread on the bed. That sort of thing may have reduced the risk of deep vein thrombosis, which we now know was increased by all that enforced bed rest.

Poor housing had serious effects on women's health. To keep the houses and children clean and free from bugs required a huge effort, especially when there was no running water. Edie M. describes the conditions that contributed to her first baby's death from gastroenteritis in the very hot summer of 1921:

> I only ever had one room to live in for a very, very long time. At that particular time, we were living with his mother over in Stepney. They had a Coronation Street house, two up, two down, and about six or seven kids. We were in one tiny little room. We had a little backyard with freezing cold water. I used to go out there and do me bit of washing.
>
> After a very bad time in that house (I'd lost one baby and I was now pregnant), my mother-in-law committed suicide, over poverty. She got into such a lot of debt, she took carbolic acid. Oh, I tried to mind her kids what were my in-laws. He had a paper stall, the father did. He was a dear old boy, and he used to bring home half-a-crown a day to keep his family. Well, I've always been very clean and that house was bug-ridden – millions and millions of them behind every picture. So I started cleaning up, burning this, burning that. And filthy heads they all had. I learnt how to clean – let's put it plain – lousy heads and get rid

of bugs. I soaked them in paraffin for a few hours, then washed it off. I had all them children's lousy heads to clean up but I got rid of them.

The daughter, Nellie, must have been about twelve, just old enough to resent me taking over. One night my father-in-law said to me, 'Edie, would you mind if Nellie takes over? She's upset about you burning things'. 'Not a bit', I said.

I moved back to Islington to a much nicer, bigger room and my father-in-law used to bring the children over to see me but then he got ill with cancer and they were all put in a home and that all broke up...

Looking back it was a horrible life. At that time I used to always accept it because we knew no other way. We never knew carpets or fridges...

Edie's descriptions of her living situation are in stark contrast to those of Vera W., a middle-class woman of similar age:

I had a dear little bungalow in the 1930s. It was lovely, leading down to the sea front, very nice, very easy to run. There was electricity and I had a nice little gas stove. Oh yes, yes, yes. I can remember putting the nappies into a steel bucket – it would be a steel bucket – onto the gas stove to boil. And of course, we had a bathroom. Yes, yes, oh, it was quite modern in those ways.

The midwives we talked with had vivid memories of homes they had visited in this period. Some were sympathetic to the problems of poverty and inadequate housing. Elizabeth C., a working-class woman and district midwife for many years in Battersea, recalls:

Most homes I went to were sort of working-class. You know, homes where they looked for their clothes in the morning to see if the rats had taken them down under the floorboards. And you daren't go out to the toilet or anything in the night-time cause there'd be rats in it. That was after the war, too, not long ago. Somebody once said that all the babies in London on district are delivered onto the *News of the World* – I says 'They are not!' Anyway, the *News of the World* is sterile ink; printed paper is sterilized with the ink mixture.

If they hadn't got things, well, you raked round and found them. Often you came home and took your own sheets off the bed because they hadn't got any.

Elsie K., working in Derby in the 1930s, also remembered the dirt and bugs in the homes she visited:

> The conditions were very bad. Filthy, some of the back streets. They've all been demolished now. Very bad. If there was time, we used to wipe over the tops of the furniture before we laid our things out, but sometimes there was only just time to catch the baby and that was all – it never seemed to do any harm. They were used to their own germs. We used to put our coats down on newspaper to try and keep the bugs and whatnot off them.

In this and the preceding chapters, we have portrayed working conditions of both handywomen and midwives in the first half of this century. Then and now, there is abundant evidence that maternal and infant mortality and morbidity are directly related to poverty and its trappings of lack of education, frequent pregnancies, overwork, poor living conditions and poor nutrition.[5,6] Overall, there have been vast improvements in living and working standards since the days described by Edie M. in this chapter, with an ensuing improvement in mortality statistics. However, infant deaths are still more common in working-class households: poverty still causes hardship, ill-health and bereavement for childbearing women in Britain today.[7]

References

1. Cited in Kenner, Charmian, *No Time For Women*, Pandora Press, London, 1985.
2. *Woman's Own*, 1st issue, 15 October 1932.
3. *Weldon's Dressmaker*, 1932.
4. *Woman's Own*, 15 October 1932.
5. Lewis, Jane, *The Politics of Motherhood*, Croom Helm, London, 1980.
6. Thunhurst, Colin, *It Makes You Sick – The Politics of the NHS*, Pluto Press, London, 1982, pp.32–33.
7. *ibid*, p.15.

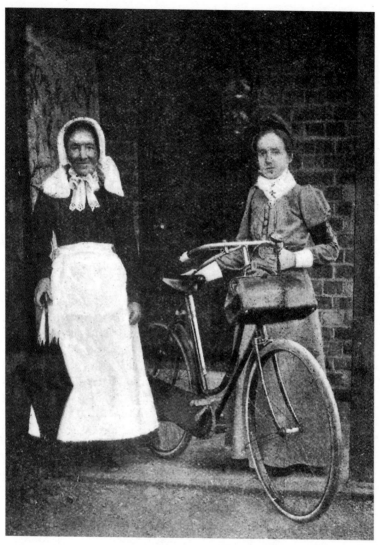

Midwives before and after the
1902 Act: a handywoman, left,
with a new professional midwife

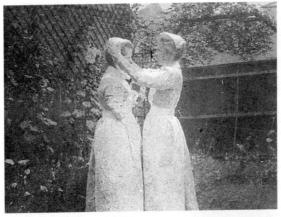

Alice Gregory and Lelia Parnell in the garden of the midwifery school they founded in 1905

Opposite: Newly born babies at Guy's Hospital, 1947, top; matron instructs mothers at a private nursing home, 1944

Lelia Parnell, hospital founder, lectures students at the British Hospital for Mothers and Babies in Woolwich

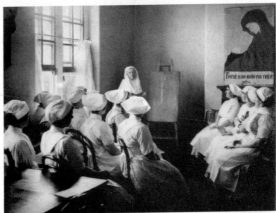

'A Little Bit of Heaven re-visited': beds on the British Hospital veranda

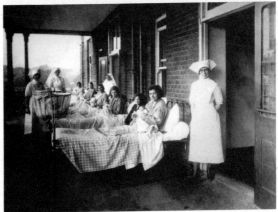

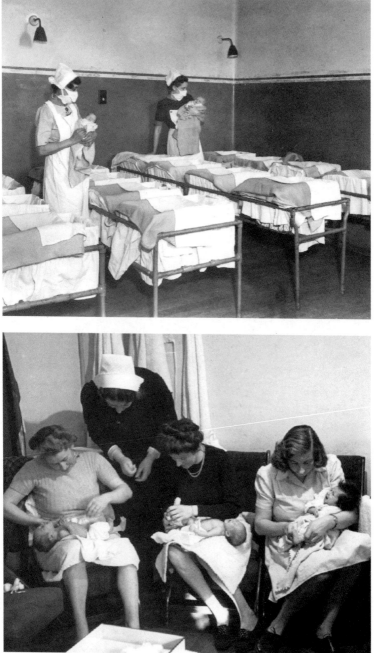

The birth of Janet at home, 31 August 1946

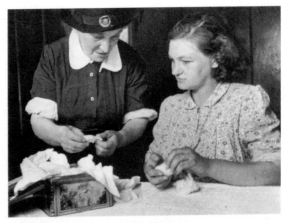

The midwife demonstrates how to pack gauze swabs in a tin; these will be sterilised by baking before the birth

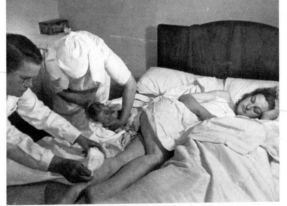

Janet is born; her mother is lying in the left lateral position much favoured by midwives at the time

Below: the midwife attends to the baby

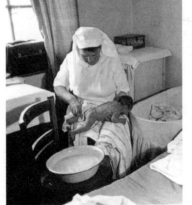

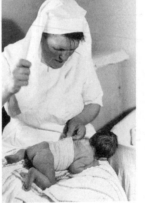

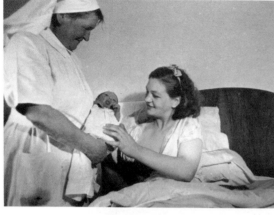

The midwife hands
Janet back to her
mother

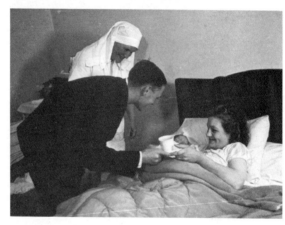

Janet's father is
allowed to meet the
new baby

Janet is shown to
her siblings

A midwife leaves for work in Deptford, South London, 1946

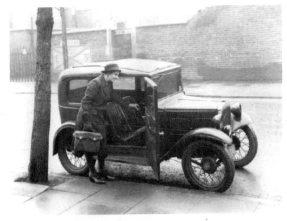

The midwife hands over care of the mother and her baby to the health visitor

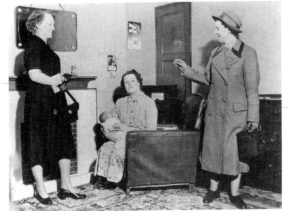

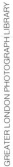

Opposite: Midwife working in a rural area, 1942

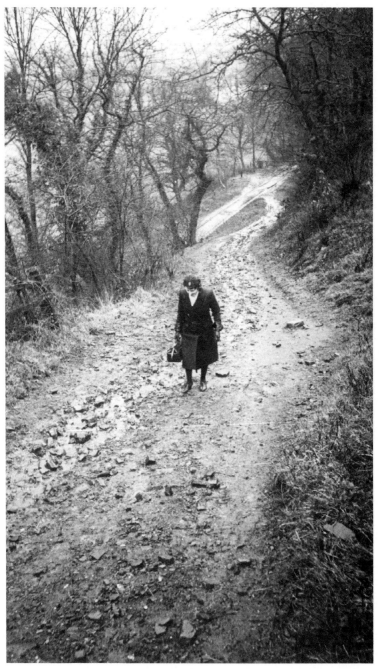

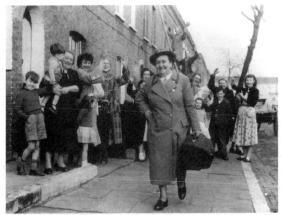

Elsie Walkerdine on her retirement in 1957

Below:
Handywoman
Mrs G., 1989;
Esther S., 1940;
Mary W., 1931

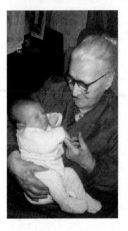
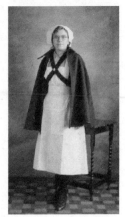
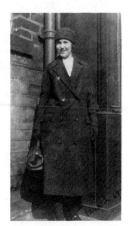

Right: Katherine L. and Margaret A. 'on the district' in 1967

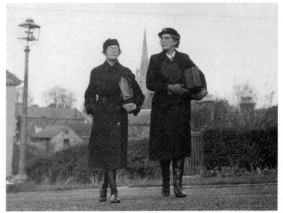

10 The experience of birth: women tell their stories

You had all sorts of funny things happen...

In pre-NHS days, most births took place at home. Either a midwife, a handywoman or maybe a doctor would be present (or perhaps even a combination of all three).[1] Mollie T., a retired midwifery tutor who worked on the district in Bermondsey in the 1940s, explains what she thinks were the reasons that women had their babies at home:

> Thinking of the poverty – and people were so poor – I was thinking of the reasons why people stayed at home. In the lower social group, I don't think it was anything emotional at all as we now know it. They hadn't got night clothes and although hospitals issued them they didn't want it known. They also had communal washing things at home, one face flannel, one toothbrush and they didn't want to show that one up either. They had to stay at home because husband would drink or gamble or bring another woman home, children wouldn't be fed, there was no home-help service, they wanted to go back to work. This still happens – in certain parts of the country with early transfers, you'd be best to check the strawberry fields before calling at home. The other thing was – and still is again now – that the husband couldn't afford to take time off work for fear of losing his job.
>
> I think the middle classes at about the same time were unable to afford a nursing home and couldn't visualise themselves mixing in hospitals. In many of the public hospitals, the maternity ward was in fact the workhouse and nobody wanted that. In fact, the care there was often superior to the nursing homes if they did but know it. These middle classes had a very great personal insecurity

for they'd been brought up in the bosom of the family and went from that to marriage and had never really been on their own. To be separated was quite devastating. This was an aspect of hospital care that I found repeated over the years even in general nursing.

Some of the upper classes would have been to boarding school and so were much more resilient and self-reliant. They had no desire to be contaminated by mixing with the lower classes. They would employ a private monthly nurse and as a pupil I did get one or two gilt-edged deliveries in a rather fashionable part of the town because the woman got on rather quickly and then the monthly nurse took over. When we were called in an emergency, they were often surprised to find we were clean and quite educated; and later welcomed us back as visitors.

By the late 1940s, the home birth rate had decreased to about 50 per cent[2] and many people were beginning to see hospital birth as superior. Midwife Elizabeth C. notes:

Nowadays, most women have their babies in hospital whether they like it or not, don't they? You nearly have to fight to have your baby at home. *Before*, you nearly had to fight to get into hospital. Just after the war, I had one young chap, he was blazing mad. He said, 'If I hadn't bothered getting married and we'd just had a baby, my wife would have got into hospital'. He said, 'Just because we're married she has to have it at home'.

In pre-NHS days, most middle-class women who could afford to pay the fees opted for giving birth in private hospitals or nursing homes. Otherwise, hospital beds were reserved only for women who were considered 'at risk' obstetrically. The cost of such beds would be subsidised by either the local authority, charitable institutions or insurance schemes. Giving birth in hospital certainly did not mean that women received better care, either physically or emotionally. Hannah H. remembers the birth of her first daughter in London in 1928:

It was a long labour; it was all night and a part of a day. They just put you in a room and let you be done with it. They used to say, 'Don't bear down, bear down, do this, do that'. They didn't used to take you into the labour room till the waters broke. But if your waters broke early and you were still not getting the baby, you stayed in the labour room anyway. And it was very bad – I think they used forceps for her because she was bruised each side of her head when I had her. Nobody with me, only the nurse sitting there. She said, 'Oh, the next one won't be so bad'. I didn't have any painkillers, I don't even think I had a smeller, did I? Didn't have anything to smell. Maybe I did, but I don't remember; it was so long ago.

In both home and hospital settings, births were essentially 'natural': women usually laboured without painkillers or medical intervention. Midwives were only allowed to give very mild painkillers and sedatives, such as potassium bromide and chloral hydrate. From 1936, they were allowed to use 'gas and air' machines, which provided mild pain relief during labour. However, strong analgesics such as chloroform were only used by doctors.[3]

The 'natural' births of pre-NHS days were a far cry from 'natural childbirth' as it is thought of today. Women usually knew little about their bodies, which would make the process of giving birth very frightening. Birth was viewed as an extremely painful event and there was no expectation of it being an emotionally fulfilling experience. This attitude was true for all the women that we interviewed, including the midwives. Ruby C. remembers giving birth to her first baby in Belfast in October 1918:

> Oh God, I thought, this is the end of the world. I kept praying all the time. 'Oh, this is terrible, I'll never get through this.' And the doctor – oh, he was lovely – he kept stroking me – 'You'll be all right, dear, no, don't you worry'. He was a bit easy-going, you know. Ay, he stroked my head – 'It's going to be all right, dear, and you'll forget about this in a very short time'. And it's true, childbirth, you do forget, don't you? I think it's nature's way, or you'd never have any more!

Births were very much 'managed' by the helpers present, with the midwives and doctors disinfecting and sterilising and generally attempting to create a mini-hospital within the home. 'Delivering' was the key word: the woman was 'delivered' of her baby by the birth attendant whose job was to organise everything and to tell the woman exactly what to do. Today in Britain, a 'woman-led' concept of choice and empowerment for women in childbirth is advocated even at government levels,[4] but attitudes such as those described by Ruby C. still prevail:

You weren't allowed to walk around. I was walking around
and the doctor came like and 'Oh, get into bed, get into bed!'
You weren't allowed to have a baby like you'd want to have
it. I think this new method's the best where they're allowed
to sit up or stand up, or run around [laughs] with the baby
hanging out! Oh Lord, sounds a bit ridiculous! But they
made you lie down on the old iron bed. They bossed you
around. Oh, it was 'Agony Ivy!' [laughs]

Poverty and birth

In the 1930s, the unemployment level was between 20 and 25 per
cent. It was estimated that one third of the population was
suffering from serious dietary deficiencies, and one half was too
poor to buy an adequate diet.[5]

Edie M.'s third baby had cerebral palsy. She has spent a lifetime
wondering if her poor diet could have been a contributing factor
to his disability:

David was born later in life, weren't he? It was 1935 and I
would have been 33 years old. I was still living in one
room but this time over in my sister's house in Dulwich.
Fine healthy chap, picture of a boy but he's spastic. I've often
wondered what caused it. I've got a funny feeling his
trouble could have been down to my diet...

I was under a clinic in Southampton Street in Peckham
and you went down there to have a check up every now and
then. I was down there for me usual. I was lying on the table
and I heard the man that was doing the talking to these
students saying, 'Now, this is what we would call a *poor*
patient'. I jumped up and he said, 'I don't mean in clothes
or money, I mean in feeding'. I was lying there with no
clothes on so it had nothing to do with me outside clothes.
It must have showed on me body. 'You have plenty of
pudding and two veg. and potatoes, do you?' he says.
'Yeah...', I says. 'Ah, but you don't get a lot of fruit, do you?'
'No, never have fruit, we can't afford it'.

But they got it wrong 'cause they said I would go another
month. No, listen to this bit. I had that checkup that day
at the clinic and I went home. That night I went to bed and
I began to get pain. I thought, 'I've got a cold in my
tummy. I've only been to the clinic today and they said I've
got another month to go'. Later, they said, 'But you've had
a family, you must have known you were in labour'. But I

said, 'I didn't. They told me I had another month to go and I didn't want to make meself look silly'.

I had a different thing in that birth that I never had before. I sat about, wrapped in a blanket, losing water. We had burst pipes in the house and the joke in the house was, 'The only one who's got any water is Edie!'

Suddenly I said, 'Alec, quick, go down and get Em' (that's my sister). I said, 'I think the baby's coming'. He jumped out of bed and she sent him off to get the nurses. I was walking about and I said, 'Oh I think it's coming Em!' She said, 'Well, get on the bed'. So I did and the baby shot out and she just covered me over. 'Lay still', she says, 'Won't be a minute'. You see, nothing was done for that baby. She didn't handle nothing. Us sisters were like that. If it had been her, I would have probably covered her over rather than touch the baby. Perhaps today, with a little bit more knowledge I might have done something?...

I lay there, ten minutes, quarter of an hour – I don't know the time, you lose count – then Alec came back with the nurse. Well, whether it happened then, while he was lying there or whether it was because he was a month beforehand I don't know...

Of course, it could have been something else. I went to put my head in the oven one night. My husband had been out all night and was drunk again and I was having another baby. Well, I was half gassed and then pulled out, opened all the windows, hysterical...

The consultant, a big man, said, 'Extreme worry or too quick a birth', but I can't think that worry done it because I had a friend that had a terrific lot of worry and she had a fine baby. I've often wondered...

When I think what's going to happen to my David, I have to try and block it out. 'Now stop it, Edie, stop it'. David says, 'I hope you live to be a hundred, Mum'. I says, 'I hope so, love. Let's do our best.'

It is impossible to tell which of the factors outlined by Edie might have been responsible for David's cerebral palsy, although recent research suggests that in most cases, the damage is caused during the pregnancy, not labour.[6]

Edie's story highlights the fact that in those days, working-class women often went into labour undernourished, tired and anxious. For those with children, another baby often meant more stress on top of an already intolerable situation. Apart from the physical hazards of bearing many children, women also faced the enormous worry of another mouth to feed, another body to clothe and another potential source of bereavement.

High infant and child mortality rates meant that women could not afford to be sentimental about their children. Molly and Lily, two sisters who grew up on Tyneside in the 1920s, discuss this:

> Death and poverty and hunger were just accepted. There wasn't a lot of sentimentality around. I can't ever remember seeing Auntie Jane or anybody weeping or wailing [about their babies' deaths]. But whether they wept in private? Perhaps they did in private but it was never outwardly. (*Lily*)
>
> No, no, I can't ever remember my mum hugging me. I can't ever remember her putting her arms around me – *never*. I mean, she had so many. I don't know – never kissed you, did she?... I can't remember any of them around there showing affection. It was considered a 'display', a silly thing, you didn't do that sort of thing, you just didn't do it. I think it's sort of brushed off on Lily and I. We don't kiss much. We were brought up not to show affection. I think it's a shame, a great shame. (*Molly*)
>
> But I don't think she loved us any the less for it. She was a good mother, she really was... (*Lily*)

Mortality

Whether a woman was poor or well off, each birth brought with it the potential threat of death for both the baby and the mother. Although infant mortality rates fell steadily throughout the 1930s, neonatal mortality (deaths within the first four weeks of life) did not.[7] Maternal mortality actually rose, so that about 3,000 women died every year in England and Wales from child-bearing or related conditions. Morbidity rates (deterioration in women's health as a result of pregnancy and birth) were also appallingly high. For example, in 1931, it was estimated that at least 60,000 women – 10 per cent of all mothers – were more or less crippled as the result of childbearing.[8]

Handywomen working in the early 1900s would have been all-too-familiar with women dying in childbirth. Mrs G., however, did not wish to be drawn into discussion on the subject:

Of course, I've seen them die. I've seen them die with the baby half out and half in. Couldn't stay that way, could it, so you had to bring it away and that was it. Well, you expect that sort of thing, don't you? You got to take it as it happens. Sometimes the women died of exhaustion, you see, because they're frightened. They're frightened to bear down in case it's going to split something. You can understand it really. But I don't think so many dies in childbirth as what they makes out.

Midwives working on the district rarely saw women die because, on the whole, they would transfer to hospital any women with severe problems. Esther S.'s only experience of a maternal death on the district was clearly a death due to a complicated hospital birth:

I did have one woman who died. It wasn't *my* delivery. One of those that came out from St. Mary's. She'd had twins that died. She was very toxic [suffering from septicaemia, blood poisoning] when she came home and I wasn't at all happy with her. Unfortunately, I had an older doctor who didn't respond. She was an embolism in the end. I reported it in the morning and the doctor thought it was a form of pleurisy bronchitis. I went again in the evening and told my supervisor I was concerned about this patient...and the next morning she was dead; she just died.

No other maternal deaths. Of course, we got stillborns but only very rarely fresh stillborns. Mine all died from abnormalities. But you don't think along these lines, do you. You must think on perfect lines.

Mary T. remembers her friend, Elsie Walkerdine, transferring a women in labour who subsequently died:

I know Elsie took a girl in once to Greenwich – St. Alfreges Hospital, it was then. It was her first baby. I don't know, Elsie told whoever was in charge what was going on. And Elsie wasn't very happy about what happened. When Elsie took her in, they should have given her a Caesarean, or whatever. But they didn't, and the girlie died. It wasn't the same day. If it was the same day, you might say, 'Oh, midwife took her in too late' – but it wasn't the same day. And Elsie said she should never have died. As far as I know, out of over 4,000 births, Elsie never had any maternal deaths.

Births with risk factors

It would be wrong to suggest that midwives in pre-NHS days only dealt with straightforward cases at home. Midwives describe breeches, twins, triplets, and women with complicated medical and obstetric histories – all giving birth at home, usually with the midwife as the sole attendant. Margaret A. tells a story that would make today's birth attendants shudder:

> I had a girl once who had twins – boy twins. They were six or seven pounds each, and she was a fortnight overdue. Now that girl had had a placenta praevia [the placenta situated across the cervix – a situation that would be life-threatening for both mother and baby] three years previously for which she'd gone into our little local general cottage hospital here for a Caesarean. And three years later she carried twins a fortnight overdue – and she was left at home to have them. One was a breech. It came out very easily. You know, I've sometimes gone cold when I think about it. No doctor there, just me.

Many women with risk factors invariably refused to go into hospital – for example, those who had had many babies before. 'Grand multipara' [or grand multip] is the name given to a woman having her fourth, or subseqent baby, and today she would be firmly advised not to opt for home birth as there could be serious obstetric complications during labour. Midwives working 50 years ago seemed to take grand multiparas in their stride, as Mary T. bears witness:

> I went with her when she [midwife Elsie Walkerdine] had that 21st baby in Deptford High Street. She woke me up this particular night and said, 'I'm going out, Mary'. I said, 'Oh, all right, Elsie, where are you going?' So she said, 'Mrs B.' 'Ooh', I said, 'I must come and see this one!' So I went and saw her 21st baby born. Of course, it took all the calorie out of her having all them babies. She looked very thin. But the birth was no bother.

Esther S. will never forget attending a woman having her 13th baby:

> We delivered the grand multips at home, then, and you know – the funniest thing! I delivered a baby, the 13th baby, funnily enough, in Portsmouth, and you know when the

placenta turns inside out, they call it the 'Matthew Duncan' form of expulsion after some obstetrician who wrote about it years ago. And I said, 'Oh, a Matthew Duncan!' And she said, 'Oh, is that what I've got then?' So I said, 'what do you mean?' She said, 'Here's you naming the baby – he's Matthew Duncan. Oh, I like those names'. She called her baby that – it's true! The 13th baby, so she had a game to know what she was going to call it, probably. So I named that baby Matthew Duncan! [laughter] Good, wasn't it?!

Elizabeth C. was one of the many midwives who told us stories of women who refused to go into hospital:

We said to this woman, 'You'll have to go into hospital for X-ray and so on, you're having twins'. She said, 'I don't want to'. Doctor says, 'Well, you might die at home'. She says, 'If I'm going to die, I'll die at home'. And she didn't die. It's just as normal as having one, having two – a bit more risk of bleeding – but not much extra risk if gently handled.

Unlike today, it was considered 'normal' to have breeches and twins at home. Nellie H. talked calmly of a twin birth that would shock midwives today who are taught that twins must be delivered in hospital and that, in the interests of safety, the second twin must be born within 20 minutes of the first:

I did get one girl that had twins and she had one twin one night and the next twin 24 hours later, and she was quite happy and she didn't want to go into hospital – I knew she was all right. I knew the twins were situated well and that it would come when it was ready – so why worry?! But now they shove them into hospital and half the time I think they die from overtreatment.

Midwives such as Esther S. spoke with pride about the twin deliveries they had attended at home:

I've had six sets of twins at home. I've had a wonderful association with them all. I've kept up with them, been to their weddings. Just been to one set of twins – their mum's funeral. I used to get letters when they'd passed their 11 plus [exam] and all that business. 'Dear Nurse, I thought you'd like to know that Robert has passed his 11 plus. I knew you were always interested in him'. Things like that – lovely. Ever so many weddings.

Elsie B. remembers triplets being born at home:

> We had one lot of triplets, I must say there was a doctor
> there. That was a woman who'd been into the nursing
> home for her first two babies and the next one she stayed
> at home. After that we couldn't get her in! She had triplets
> and two sets of twins at home and she'd had the first two
> single births in the nursing home! No, you had all sorts of
> funny things happen...
>   There's so much said about 'the risk' and all the rest, that
> you frighten a lot of the people. There's things that in the
> old days would never enter their minds that could happen
> to them. Well, they were happy. And you can think things
> will happen and then they will happen. There isn't the
> patience these days.

Elsie Walkerdine obviously did not consider it necessary to
call out the doctor to a triplet birth, as her friend Mary T.
remembers:

> I remember when she had triplets down Hyde Street. She
> never called the doctor in till after. So he says, 'Sister, you
> should have let me in on this' (that was Dr R-J. in Edward
> Street). So she says, 'Why? What for?' She says, 'There was
> nothing wrong. It was all straightforward. If I'd have
> called you in, I would have frightened the patient'. Three
> girls they were.

Midwives spoke of Caesarean sections as rarities in the first half
of the century. Nowadays, the Caesarean section rate in some
London teaching hospitals is between 15 and 20 per cent and the
forceps rate aproximately 7 to 10 per cent. So it is awe-inspiring
to hear midwives like Bronwen H. talk of their work in the mid-
1920s:

> I only had to call a doctor to do forceps about four or five
> times, and only one Caesarean section in 200 births when
> I was on the district. I didn't have to send anyone in. I
> always considered myself lucky.

Lucky indeed! The only Caesarean that she was involved in was
a home birth. Bronwen explained how, in 1926, she and the G.P.
(who was later to become her husband) were called to a woman in
labour who refused to go into hospital even though she needed a
Caesarean as the baby was too big to fit through her pelvis:

She wouldn't go in! You see...it's...it's hard to explain. It's difficult when you don't know anything about the people. I mean, I'd only seen to her about once, you see. Didn't know anything about her. She just couldn't be persuaded to go in.

Of course, my husband, he was a bit nervous doing the Caesarean in the house and thought, 'Oh dear...' Anyway, I thought, 'I wonder if she'll be all right'. You know, the risk of infection – no antibiotics or anything in those days.

Anyway, we did it on the kitchen table and I arranged with the people downstairs that when the baby was born I'd bang on the floor with a broom so that they could come up and take care of the baby, you see. So anyway, we did the Caesarean in this room, everything according to plan, and somebody came up and took the baby down. I said, 'Keep it warm but not too near the fire and don't leave it on the side'. So we finished off the mother and packed her up, and then I did the baby. Well, everything went according to plan. A *beautiful* boy about 8lbs! And you know, she was only about 4 foot 11.

Anyway, everything went according to plan and in about a fortnight's time the wound had healed and I found the baby wasn't putting on weight. So I told her how to feed the baby and all that sort of thing. Well, in a day or two she had mastitis, then an abscess. Now we didn't know much about that then. In those days it was lancing that was the thing, you see. Then the pus poured out.

Anyway, she got over that all right, so I attended her for a month and saw that she was all right and then I said, 'Now I'm not coming any more, but I'll call in a few days to see how you are'.

So I called in a few days and she and her husband had flown, with the baby. They hadn't even paid the lady the rent. So anyway, about a couple of months after that, the police came to talk to me and my husband about them. Anyway, we discovered eventually that they'd moved to the Midlands from Wales and the reason the police came to see us was the police in the Midlands wanted to know all about them. Apparently, they took two rooms and then one day they said they were going to see about buying a house and would she look after the baby until they came back. So the lady of course looked after the baby and then the parents never turned up!

We discovered afterwards that he was somebody else's husband... I felt very sorry for her really because she must have been in dreadful agony, I should think. I don't know what happened to the baby – probably it was put out for adoption. We didn't know, didn't hear any more about it. Oh, it was very sad.

One of the women we interviewed, Alice F. described having a timely Caesarean section in 1937. She spoke with pride about the experience:

I went into hospital, and I had to wait and wait. Three times I went into false labour and that was horrific. I don't know if you know labour pains? You do – well, they're murder, aren't they?! And then, of course, they kept on putting needles in my botty to bring on the false labour – no painkillers. On the third attempt, I thought I was going to get the baby but I heard the doctor – he swore – he said, 'This child is determined to come standing up...' Afterwards, as I told you, they reckoned there was a piece of bone right across and the baby couldn't get out. And, of course, he was a big baby for little me. I'm not big now, but I was very slim when I got married. I only had a 19-inch waist.

And so the baby was born and I was all worried – 'Was it perfect?' You know, and all that. Caesarean, of course. I've still got the wotsit down there. Well, he was beautiful. One mass of thick curly hair, black, bright blue eyes. The Sister was very, very pleased. She said 'I'm very, very pleased about this birth because it's so beautiful and clean'. She said 'You must have drunk castor oil by the bottle'. And I had! 'Cause we had a nurse there and she was rather strict, and she said, 'If you don't take this castor oil, I shall hold your nose and pour it down you'. I said, 'You don't have to, Nurse, I've been drinking it even before I came in here'. 'Let me see you do it then'. And I drunk it right down. The Sister said to me 'It was the most beautiful birth, I'm very, very pleased with it'.

As with Caesarean sections, the midwives spoke of forceps deliveries as rare and implied that people these days lack the skill of patience – '*We* waited for them [the babies] to come'. Elsie B. remembers:

I'm not saying we never did do them. Well, I didn't, but you helped the doctor. Then they used to use a little chloroform on a mask. I've given chloroform on the mask numbers of times, when you got stuck like that. We did them at home because you didn't have enough beds in hospitals to send all these people in there.

Although the comparatively high number of instrumental deliveries today is being questioned, there is another side to the coin. In the past, without easy access to hospital facilities, many women laboured on until their babies died. The doctor and midwife then had the gory and disturbing job of dismembering the baby and crushing its skull in order to remove it vaginally. There was a high risk of infection and, in the days before antibiotics, many women died. Bronwen H. spoke with distress of being involved in such a delivery in Wales:

In the beginning of September 1927 we had a case – a tiny little woman. She hadn't booked anybody. One of my mothers that I was attending said to me, 'Oh, Mrs H., she's expecting, has she booked you, Nurse?' I said, 'No'. 'Well', she said, 'If I were you I should go and have a look at her'.

So being nosy, I went to have a look at her. And honestly, when I saw her I said, 'Well, when is your baby due?' 'Oh', she said, 'In about two weeks' time'. I said, 'Well, have you booked a nurse or a doctor?' 'No', she said, 'I haven't'. 'Well,' I said, 'I think you'd better book a doctor'.

So anyway I sent this note down to the doctor and in a day or two she started labour. But her membranes had ruptured some time before and the baby wouldn't come through. So, anyway, the doctor came up and we had to do a craniotomy. But fortunately the baby had died because... Oh, I don't know...it was a funny affair really. Husband was more or less a cripple and a mother's boy and she, poor dear... Anyway, I attended her for about a month and she got on like a top. Not even a whisper of a temperature or anything. It was interesting but *very* upsetting.

But I think they were thrilled to think the baby hadn't lived. They were glad it was dead because...well, they *had* to get married in the beginning. And there was all this fuss with the mother-in-law and oh, I don't know... One doesn't know half the things that go on with these people.

The funny part about it, a few years afterwards when I was married and had children of my own, I was driving along the road and I saw her pushing a pram with four little ones with her. One tiny little toddler hanging onto

her...and the mother wasn't much taller than the pram!
And I thought, 'Well, really...!'

Stillbirth at home

Esther S. spoke from personal experience about the lack of
knowledge about appropriate support around stillbirths in pre-NHS
days:

> I lost my first baby. He was a fresh stillbirth. Of course, I
> was devastated. I was very shocked about it all – you can
> imagine, can't you?
>
> You never forget these things – all the little details. I'd
> put out all the best clothes for my baby to air on the
> clothes horse. I had him dressed for burial in all those best
> clothes. In those days, they were disposed of in this horrible
> cardboard box – I used to have to go and get it myself later
> in my work – terrible isn't it?
>
> When I went back to work some time later, something
> happened that made me think, 'These things are meant to
> be...' I had to go and do 'nursings' [postnatal visits] in a new
> area – because of course I'd had to give up my old area when
> I got pregnant – and the first one I went to, that baby was
> exactly the same weight as my baby had been – five pounds
> – and he had exactly the same look – fair, he was a very fair
> child. So I thought, 'That's exactly what my baby would
> have looked like if he'd lived. So I picked him up, cuddled
> him and cried over him. And then I thought, 'Now I can
> do it'.
>
> In those days, you see, they didn't know about letting you
> hold them when they died, they just didn't know. And I
> was so distraught and didn't know to ask. It was devastat-
> ing for my friend who was my midwife, too.
>
> But I do think that with an experience like that, you're
> better off at home. You haven't got to come back into
> your home and enter it. You're with people, you know.
> Nowadays, of course, they know much more about how to
> help people through it with the aftercare and counselling.
> But it's a very traumatic thing. So is miscarriage. I had one
> of them after that before I had my two children. Those expe-
> riences are with you all your life...

Premature births

Prior to the 1950s, babies born prematurely were usually cared for
at home. Certainly, very small babies did survive without the use
of incubators. They would have had carefully improvised circumstances, such as those described to us by Katherine L. and
Margaret A., sisters who worked together in East Anglia in the
1940s:

> Oh, we had a wonderful premature baby! One Sunday
> morning, we were just getting our dinner. There was snow
> on the ground and along came a worried relative. 'Nurse,
> can you come quickly, one of the girls has just had a baby?'
> He didn't say what. He didn't say how.
>
> Well, round we went. And the poor little baby was 10
> weeks prem. and had been born in the latrine, the outside
> loo, down the bottom of the garden. She'd lived with her
> sister, who didn't know she was pregnant. She was com-
> plaining of stomach-ache, poor Mary, so her sister gave her
> a whopping dose of castor oil – and poor Mary went and
> had it in the loo! And a neighbour came along – I'll always
> remember it – and two men on either side of Mary
> manhandled her into the house and old Mrs Auger (the
> handywoman) came along holding the baby in her hands,
> up the garden path and up the stairs. It weighed about two
> and a half pounds and it was just like a plum to look at,
> wasn't it. And the doctor said, 'You can't wish that on the
> matron (in the cottage hospital). Do what you can for it.'
>
> And so we cleared a room downstairs and put a bed in
> it. We turned our house inside out, didn't we, Kath? We
> loaned them all sorts of things: we loaned them a Moses
> basket, a bedside lamp, an electric blanket, two little electric
> pads that Dad had given us – everything we could think of!
> We came home and made premature baby clothes out of
> white lint and we reared that baby inside that room. We
> had great big notices on the door – 'NO ADMITTANCE
> EXCEPT IN EMERGENCY'. And we were the only ones
> allowed in there, and Mary, of course. Nobody was allowed
> to go in there without a mask on. They had to wash their
> hands and put a gown and a mask on.

The baby was too small to breast-feed, but Mary had masses of milk so we used to express the milk and feed the baby with a 'Belcroy' – the 'Belcroy' is like a very small glass tube. It has one big bulb on one end and a tiny little teat on the other and you put that little teat in the baby's mouth and you press the bulb and it literally squirts it down the baby. It doesn't have to work very hard to get it. We gave it a few tube feeds of breast milk, too.

The baby gained weight rapidly. It did ever so well and when it should have been born, it was a normal birth weight and then Mary's milk went! It weighed seven and a half pounds and the milk dried up!

Mary was a young, single girl. She had a boyfriend who lived there with them. And they got married before the time was up that the baby had to be registered...and she went along and she was 'churched' [reference to 'the Churching of Women', a Christian service of thanksgiving and 'purification' for women who have recently given birth].

Of course, she had been keeping quiet about being pregnant because she was going to look after her sister, Edna, who was expecting her own baby in ten weeks time. So then we had Edna...! They were a very nice family. The baby grew up – he's had seven lives! He was at the motor pump the other day, when we were getting filled up, and his hair's white!

But that was a feat really! That really was a most remarkable feat: to rear that baby under those circumstances, because they hadn't anything really, had they, Kath? (*Margaret A.*)

Clearly, the experience of birth in pre-NHS days presented both women and attendants with enormous challenges. Most women gave birth at home and there were surprisingly few fatalities, given the circumstances.

References

1. Towler, Jean and Bramall, Joan, *Midwives in History and Society*, Croom Helm, Beckenham, UK, 1986, Chapter 8.
2. Campbell, Rona and Macfarlane, Alison, *Where to be Born – The Debate and the Evidence*, National Perinatal Epidemiology Unit, Oxford, 1987, p.12.
3. Towler, Jean and Bramall, Joan, *op. cit*, p.222.

4. House of Commons Health Committee, *Report on Maternity Services*, HMSO, London, 1992.
5. Oakley, Ann, *The Captured Womb*, Basil Blackwell, Oxford, 1984, p.91.
6. Editorial, 'Cerebral Palsy, Intra-partum Care and a Shot in the Foot', 1989, *Lancet*, pp.1251–1252.
7. Oakley, Ann, *The Captured Womb*, Basil Blackwell, Oxford, 1984, p.87.
8. *ibid*, p.68.

11 Midwifery practice in pre-NHS days: 'the tricks of the trade'

Nature is the best way but you can aid it.

As we have seen in the last chapter, in pre-NHS days midwives were the sole practitioners at most births, including breeches and twins. Up until the late 1940s, most babies were born at home.[1] In the Yorkshire mining town where Mary W. worked, 90 per cent of the births still took place at home when she retired in 1968:

> I still think there's a lot to be said for home deliveries you know. You're so much more relaxed at home. I think on the whole they were happier at home.

Most of the material in this chapter emerged from discussions we had about what we would do in certain midwifery situations. This was often a two-way process, with all of us equally interested in comparing notes. The midwives spoke about their work with awe-inspiring confidence and many of them were disparaging about what they saw as a lack of patience and a loss of skill in present-day midwifery. Elsie K. voices a common opinion:

> They didn't have so many Caesars then. One of my friends wrote to me last week of how her daughter had had a baby and they'd done a Caesar because it was a face presentation – well, I've delivered a face presentation without any need for a Caesar. They do Caesars very easily these days. They've lost the old skills, they're more slapdash today.

As discussed in Chapter 3, until the 1936 Midwives Act made it mandatory for local supervising authorities to provide a salaried midwifery service, most midwives were on call 24 hours a day with little, if any, 'off duty'. This system may have been exhausting for the midwives, but it did mean that most women benefited from total continuity of care from their midwife. Until well into the 1930s, however, the focus of midwifery care was on the labour and postnatal visiting, rather than on the antenatal period.

Antenatal care

The concept of preventative antenatal care was one that grew slowly in Britain and was applied variably until well after the Maternal and Child Welfare Act of 1918 encouraged local authorities to set up antenatal clinics. In the first decades of the century, midwives tended to visit the women at home in early pregnancy to make arrangements for the birth, but thereafter, would only see her if an obvious problem arose in the pregnancy. In such a case, the woman would be referred to a doctor. Sissy S. from Deptford, has no memory of receiving antenatal care during her pregnancies in the 1920s and 1930s, although she remembered some contemporary advice:

> If you was anaemic, you was advised to take a bottle of stout or Guinness. But sometimes the nurse would send you to the doctor to get a tonic.

Mollie T. describes another, somewhat curious, initiative that was set up in an attempt to combat anaemia:

> I think the reason for the low haemoglobins in the locality was in the industrial activity, and the women had a strong reluctance to taking iron. Iron really did upset them. In this area [Bermondsey] they were so undernourished that one of the jobs the midwife used to do was to deliver egg custards to try and get concentrated protein into them. She probably baked them in the health centre or hospital kitchen, if not at home. The early training schools included a course and examination in cookery for this reason. The problems of looking after these patients hinged very much on nourishment.

Whatever methods were employed, in 1934 the Central Midwives Board Rules stated that the midwife should:

> ...make as sure as is humanly possible that no complications occur that can be foreseen and/or prevented and that no early signs of disordered function escape undetected.[2]

Despite the ruling of the Central Midwives Board, antenatal care was often not given high priority. Pregnancy was still seen as a normal process that did not need much attention. Mary W. explains:

> Antenatal care was patchy. It was left to the midwife a great deal, and you were on you own and too overworked to do it properly. I used to try to keep to a pattern, but of course, if you got a delivery, the antenatal used to be pushed aside. But we always tried to get them in. You palpated [felt the woman's abdomen to determine the baby's position, size and development] and did urine tests – that's about all. I think we got sphygs [sphygmomanometers] to do blood pressures in about '37.
>
> Some people objected to the antenatal examination. Some of them were very coy, even with the midwife. Some people thought antenatal care was all a lot of fuss.

Preparation of the room

We gained the impression from our research that whereas antenatal care was often non-existent or given low priority in the 1920s and 1930s, a great deal of emphasis was placed on preparing the room and the linen for labour. This is understandable if we consider conditions such as those in the Yorkshire mining villages described by Mary W.:

> You would tell the woman to have clean things and her bed ready, and plenty of newspaper and brown paper. And you spread it around the room, particularly round the bed. They also had to provide a mackintosh – we had a mackintosh that we could take if the woman couldn't afford one. You had to be very careful with people's belongings to see that they weren't spoiled.
>
> It was much easier once they got bathrooms. When I first started in '32, there was no pithead baths and quite a lot of the men didn't bath every day because there was this old wives' tale that bathing too much wasn't good for your back. And you'd often find half of the bed black. It was hard work for women with all the coal dust everywhere. It got everywhere. The men came home in their pit things and the women had to wash them. And then all these baby clothes, woollens and long white gowns. Terrible! No wonder they died young you know – so much work to do!

Complicated domestic arrangements were necessary for home births. Edie M. recalls her experiences in London in the 1920s:

> It was quite a performance. You had to get the room ready with enough things. A nice piece of blanket, three or four nice sheets and fresh curtains. Everything had to be ready: buckets and bowls, spotlessly clean, and some way of getting plenty of hot water. And two of everything for your baby. They used to wear body bands and vests – we dressed them different to what they do today. We'd have a penny ready to put over the navel and then bind it round. Terry towelling nappies. If you were very poor you'd only have six but I always had twelve. The reason you needed such a lot was that everything was washing in them days. No throwaway nothing, no tissues or anything. Everything was wash, wash, wash.
>
> You had your brown paper on top of the mattress, then your blanket, then your sheet – right till the end of your confinement. Then you'd take them out, burn the afterbirth in the grate and someone would make the midwife a nice cup of tea after she done her job.

Early labour

One midwife described giving quinine to start labours but others said they avoided any sort of induction of labour other than 'the occasional dose of castor oil if the woman was getting fed up with waiting'. Nellie H. had strong views about this:

> No, I didn't ever start them off, however long overdue they went. I don't think babies *are* overdue, myself. I used to wait till they started on their own. I think it's more natural.

Once a woman was in labour, the midwife would usually administer an enema and shave her pubic hair – practices that have only been phased out in the last ten years after research showed them to be unnecessary and distressing. Elsie K. describes the process:

> We always gave them enemas, unless it was too late. We used the Higginson's syringe to give enemas long before the tube and funnel. The ball was about as big as your fist and it had a piece of tubing and a nozzle, and then a rubber catheter on the end. You squeezed the ball – green soap, it

was. We used to shave the mums, too, not on the district
in the very old days but in the hospitals. After about '37 they
all had shaves. Its all gone out now, hasn't it? Well, I hope
so, I don't think it's necessary.

The progress of labour

Today, women consider themselves lucky if they have met the
midwife who attends them in labour, and luckier still if she is able
to see them through the whole process. 'Modern' obstetric practice
has dictated that the majority of women in labour are subjected
to four-hourly, or sometimes two-hourly vaginal examinations.
The results are plotted on a graph, and a high level of technology
is employed to hurry things on if there is any deviation from a
strict curve that defines so-called 'acceptable progress'. Membranes
are often ruptured routinely in early labour. Women are often not
allowed to eat and drink what they want in labour. Many women
still have a battle on their hands if they simply want to be free
to move around. Many find themselves being pressured into
accepting analgesia when they are at their most vulnerable.

Interventionist practices are a stark contrast to the methods of
early midwives. It was inspiring to listen to retired midwives
airing their views and speaking about their experiences when we
asked them to tell us how they assessed the progress of labour. Elsie
K. echoed the scorn expressed by many of the midwives regarding
today's practice of carrying out frequent vaginal examinations to
assess progress:

> We did them sometimes in labour if we felt it was required,
> but very, very seldom. We got into the habit of realising how
> the labour was progressing without a vaginal. It was quite
> easy really when you were watching the patient. I think it's
> a pity to do unnecessary internals. They shouldn't really be
> necessary in normal cases if you're keeping an eye on the
> patient. I think people rely too much on that, and too little
> on their own observations. It can't be pleasant having
> internal examinations.

Margaret A. explains further:

> Somehow or other you know, as you became more expe-
> rienced. You could just look at the patient's face and say,
> 'She's about two or three fingers [dilated]', or 'She's coming

on'. You could tell by the look on her face, not always by the number of pains she's having. You never got two alike.

Some patients are terribly bad patients, they're terribly, terribly bad. You know...they lose control and scream and carry on...and others are so relaxed and calm and quiet. But then some have a higher pain threshold than others don't they, so you can't ever be sure of how far on they are. If I could possibly stay with a patient in labour then I'd stay with them, all night if necessary. But if I was going to have to leave a patient in labour for any length of time I would always do a vaginal examination to see what was happening. If she was three or four centimetres or more, I wouldn't go. If the labour went on for hours and hours we'd do an examination to find out why, but otherwise not.

Similarly, Esther S. would only do a vaginal examination in an emergency:

> ...such as an obvious delay or if I felt the baby's heart was fluctuating – I wanted to know the reason, if it was hung up in any way... Sometimes I'd rupture the membranes but you didn't do it *ad lib.* because I think it's a good thing to have them intact. In fact, sometimes you found that if they had their membranes ruptured, they had a longer delivery. Usually they don't go till it's coming up to second stage. Then you carry on and you get a better sort of pushing then, don't you, a different sort of pushing.

On reading Alice Gregory's midwifery textbook, in which she describes the preparation considered necessary before doing a vaginal examination – sterile gloves were not in use until after 1937 – one can understand that a midwife might think twice before subjecting her hands to such a rigorous procedure:

> However necessary vaginal examinations may be, they must not be undertaken without plenty of time, and soap and water. A quarter of an hour is the least time that can be allotted for this purpose. For the preliminary bathing, three minutes' scrub of your hands, and one minute's scrub in perchloride of mercury, 1 in 1000. After the bathing, change the water; and in a full basin of clean hot water, five minutes' scrub; then a three-minute soak, and one is ready. If you have not enough time for these processes, so much the better – you have evidently not enough time to examine and the labour must be advancing rapidly.[3]

In order to be convinced that a woman was getting near to the second stage of labour, handywoman Mrs G. would have to see what she describes as 'a linking pain'. Midwives today might describe such a change in the nature of the contractions as signs of transition (transition from the first stage of labour, which is concerned with the dilating of the cervix, to the expulsive contractions of the second stage):

> I used to press their stomachs sometimes when they said there's a pain there. And I used to say, 'Well, how long have you had that pain, how long in between?' Perhaps it's an hour, perhaps it's half an hour? I'd say, 'Ooh, you've got lots more to go through first'. I'd say, 'You really must have a linking pain before you have the baby – a linking pain'. Now that's got you guessing! [laughs] A linking pain – they might call it something else now – but you have a pain and just as it's going, it comes back, you see. And then, of course, when they have a second sort of pain with the linking pain, then soon the head starts to show. I don't know whether they call it a 'linking pain' these days, do they? No, I don't suppose you've heard of it. Always have to have that linking pain. You had a double one. Just as one's going, you get another one – ooh – and it comes again.

Today, we measure dilatation of the cervix in centimetres. Previously, midwives talked about how many 'fingers' apart the cervix was. Alice Gregory, in her book, uses the coinage of the day to describe dilatation:

> 'Os from sixpence to a shilling'... 'Os a half-crown'... 'Os has reached four shillings'...and finally the exquisitively painful stage of 'lip all round', or 'edge of a teacup', as some people call it. This is the moment when a bath is a perfect godsend and I know few things which are pleasanter to do. One had to perform so many disagreeable treatments of sorts, that to drive away, or at any rate lessen, these horrible pains for half an hour and to see the patient go to sleep with her head on your knee, is really a very great pleasure.[4]

Indeed, what a shame it is that so many maternity units have ripped out the baths in favour of showers today and that there is still resistance to the use of water to ease pain in labour.

Long labours

In the long or difficult labours, hot baths could be very soothing. Esther S. extolled their virtues in helping women cope:

> I might give her another hot bath. I think that helps – you can't really quicken it up, I don't think...nature is its only best way, but you can aid. I used to rub her back because the contractions there were more severe with a posterior position [the baby lying on its back, rather than the more straightforward position of lying with its back towards the mother's abdomen]. They get more back-ache with the posteriors, don't they; very, very, painful, I believe, from what they say. And well, I just have to keep on trying to encourage her and tell her that some people do have slower labours – to see if you could put her mind at ease as well. Also, see her diet is kept up with food and drinks. They get very dehydrated if not – a very important factor. And see they empty their bladders, which is another important thing. Then you can see if there's dehydration as well [by noting the concentration of the urine].

Lou N. gives the impression that she was in control of what happened during her labours. She describes some interesting techniques for coping with a long, 'back-ache labour'.

> When you had it at home, you tied a towel round the end of your bed, then you twisted it and you pulled on it, 'cos you feel that's what you want to do. [groans] How these women want their husbands with 'em, I don't know! Blimey, I never wanted mine about the place. I just had the midwife and the woman that came in. The first one, Tommy, I had three days labour with him. Ooh! [grimaces] I started on the Saturday and I didn't have him 'till Wednesday. Blimey, he weighed 9lbs something. Oyey, he really went to town! I was married in 1931 and I had him ten months later. When I was in labour I couldn't sit still. I was moving about – I only sat down when I had to, not otherwise. Because all my pains wasn't in the stomach, they was in the back. If you were longwinded you were made to drink castor oil. Yeah, but I got the winkle of that afterwards – you put orange juice in first, and then a tiny drop of orange juice on top and that was it. It speeded you up! When I was having Joan, the old lady that was with me sent out for a great big jug of eels! She thought I had to eat hot

eels during the labour. But me, all the time I'm in there you can guess what I do – I talk, all the way through it. I talk and talk, and then when a pain come on I held on till the pain went and then I start talking again. Well, as you can guess, I've got a bad habit of talking. [laughter]

All the midwives described the virtue of getting women to walk around in labour, a practice also encouraged by 95-year-old handywoman, Mrs G:

Oh yes, we got the long labours that went on and on. Some of them were nearly a week. Well, you couldn't do nothing. Just tell 'em to walk about and that's it. Some people say, 'Lay on the bed'. But then the baby goes to sleep, doesn't it, so the mother's got to go all through that again. We used to stay with them when it started. The woman needed to know there was somebody else there.

We used to get an orange. Squeeze half into a glass, then a dessert-spoonful of castor oil, then squeeze the other half of the orange on top so they wouldn't taste the oil. That would get them going. Then they would want to go to the toilet and if the baby was there, really well down as well, you see, it was lovely, it was not much problem.

If there was something in the way, the baby wouldn't come. We used to call it 'the shutter'. It had to be lifted, you see. Until the shutter was lifted, the baby wouldn't come. You'd use your finger, see, and you had to lift it like inside. [Presumably, Mrs G. is describing lifting back a lip of cervix over the baby's head.]

When they were in real labour, they used to lay on their backs in a certain way and we used to press on their stomach, on the top of their stomach. We used to tip our hands down like that and hold the baby down a bit.

Midwife Esther S. remembered the increased pain she experienced when being forced to lie down during one of her own labours, and how that gave her insight into the benefits of what is now called 'ambulation in labour'.

We kept them moving around in labour, never went to bed until the last minute. They almost had them [the babies] standing up sometimes – 'Come on, love, on the bed. No, you can't really stay like that [mobile]'. It was lovely because they were free. There weren't all this tied down thing [reference to modern monitoring equipment]. When I went to have one of mine, I had to go into hospital for an emergency and they wouldn't let me get off the bed! I said, 'This is terrible. This is murder to me.' Terrible! Stuck where you are! Dreadful! Oh no, no, no, you want to move. Of course you do. Nature needs you to move. You let them have the freedom of what she's wanted. You got as tired as they were, you walked miles when you had deliveries!

There were times when midwives could not walk miles, since they sometimes arrived at labours exhausted from lack of sleep. Several women told stories about 'looking after the poor midwife'. Edie M., whose babies were born in the 1920s, recalls:

I called the midwife out on the Sunday. Cropped hair, proper, like a sergeant major. 'Oh you naughty girl', she said, 'Calling me out at this time. Oh, I'm ever so sorry. I've got a terrible head'. So I said, 'Lie on the couch.' 'Ooh', she says, 'Ain't it hard?!' I said, 'Well, lay on the bed'. So I put a pillow from the top to the bottom and said, 'Lay there'. And this big woman, she got on and got down. I said, 'I'll make you a nice cup of tea'. So I'm in strong labour and I'm running around! So eventually, I says, 'I'm afraid you'll have to get off. I've got to push this out!' Had to get her off to get on meself!

Margaret A. describes a similar situation, but from the midwife's point of view:

If we were at all able to stay with them in labour we did. I well remember a girl we had down the road here. She was in labour overnight. The husband came up to the house with a pair of her pants. He said, "Ere Nurse, what's that?' 'That's a show', I said. So he said, 'Well, you better come then'. So off I went. And when I got there she wasn't doing much, but obviously she'd had a show, and I thought, 'Oh well, its her sixth so I'll stay'. I gave her pot. brom. chloral and she went into a sound sleep. I got on the bed with her and I expect I dozed off as well. Slept all night. About 7 o'clock in the morning she suddenly sat up in bed and said, 'God, it's coming, Nurse!' D'you know, I didn't have time to put on me gown and me mask and me gloves! She just had it like that, slept all night and then just had it! And I had a night's rest on the bed beside her!

The pot. brom. chloral (potassium bromide chloral, or chloral hydrate) referred to by Margaret A. was a mild sedative – the only analgesic used by midwives. Even though the early gas-and-air machines (Minnitt Machines) were introduced in 1936, few midwives used them since they were too heavy and bulky to carry on foot or bicycle. Chloroform was still used occasionally at difficult deliveries, such as forceps, when the doctor had been called. Edie B. elaborates:

> We used to give them horrible stuff called chloral hydrate which used to immediately make them sick. It was no good. That was the only concession we had to pain relief then.
>
> There was one little phase where we had horrible little chloroform capsules. I don't know if anyone's told you about those? Little capsules filled with chloroform and you had a lint mask and you just squeezed one of these capsules onto the lint and put it over the patient's face every time a pain came. However, they soon stopped it because I think they found it not very successful – and a bit dangerous. [It could be fatal.] The women did begin to get a bit of relief from it, but they didn't think it was a wise thing to do, to continue with that. And, of course, when the Minnitt machine came in, that was a terrible great help... But most of the ones at home didn't want anything anyway. They moved around. They weren't restricted.

Elizabeth C.'s response to our discussion on coping with pain in labour was to emphasise the importance of continuity of care, a topical issue in midwifery today. She described accurately the release of endorphins (the body's natural opiates) in undisturbed labour, which surprised us because this process has only been given an explanation in recent years.[5]

> I'm sure it's really important to know the person who's going to look after you in labour. I've never had a baby, of course, but I'm sure it's very comforting to have someone that you know and that knows you, and sort of knows your temperament, knows what you can take and what you can't. And having a home back-up, too. Knowing the midwife, it's better than dope or something because it's a normal thing, you see.
>
> I think myself that the system has a certain amount of sedative in itself that it releases at a time like that. I'm sure

it has, because I've seen people that just looked as if they were half sozzled – and they didn't have anything! Just looked like somebody 'gone' – and they hadn't had any dope!

I think the body does release something into the system. If it's not interfered with by giving dope, it will work. But I think when you interfere, it won't work then.

Elsie B.'s tip for coping with long labours was, 'Keep them all busy and happy'. She gave this example:

One thing that happened. I think she was a primip. [first baby] All the house was very anxious and all the rest of it. So they said, 'What could they do?' So I said, 'Oh, well, keep quiet, and let her go. Sit down and have a game of cards, or do something'. When I went back and had a look in, there they all were most religiously playing cards! It worked!

The birth

Like all the women we interviewed, Sissy S. spoke vividly about each of the births of her children in the 1920s and 1930s. She remembered details as if they had happened yesterday:

You was always told to lie on your left side and 'Steady, steady…that's right – now bear down, slowly…slowly…now the next pain is going to be very hard…' ('Ooh no, the first one was bad enough!') For the head to come into the world, that was painful enough, but then you had the shoulders. After that, you might as well say it's all over. I never tore with any of my babies. Not even the one that was 12lbs. I never had a doctor to me – because if it was a tear, you had to have a doctor to you.

The midwives all talked with pride about their skills in preventing tears. Elsie K. explains:

We were taught to deliver, not just catch the baby. We were taught to guard the perineum. And it was a disgrace to get a tear. We were taught to do it properly and carefully. I know when I was a staff midwife, I was getting tears sometimes when I was delivering, so I said to the senior Sister, 'I want to watch you deliver and see what it is I'm doing wrong'. And I was really hurrying the head out a bit too much. I

watched her, you see, and realised that I must be very
much slower than I was. It's all patience in midwifery.

Elizabeth C. explains further:

You didn't have to rush things, you see. Time was not of
any great consequence. You didn't rush. Your time was your
own. You might be up all night but it was your time.

By contrast, we heard many descriptions of handywomen
getting women to bear down long before the uterus was ready to
expel the baby (a potentially harmful practice). Handywoman Mrs
G. certainly expressed a sense of urgency to 'get the baby out'. She
often implied that if the baby was not coming, it must be the
woman's fault:

And then the head comes through – that's if they lift the
shutter. Of course, if the shutter don't lift, well it's no
good is it? It's like if a person cut yer tongue out. If you cut
yer tongue out, you can't talk. That's true, isn't it? You had
to let the baby's head come through and then you held the
baby's head, and then you say, 'Well how long have you
got, mate? You gonna lay there all the time? Come on, get
cracking!' Then we used to massage the woman's stomach,
just give her a press down again. 'Come on, don't lark
about with me, that's it...'
   There was one woman, I used to laugh about her. I used
to go to her and she had four girls. And all her babies, believe
it or not, they were born hand first! So I always used to shake
their hands and say, 'You *are* polite, shaking hands first!'
They was born with their hand up alongside their heads,
you see. You wouldn't know what to do, would you? 'Cause
there's nothing you can do. If you try to push their hand
back, you might break their shoulder. All her babies came
like that – but I used to say they was polite!
   No, the women weren't always lying down, I've had
babies drop in my apron! [laughter] There used to be a lady
lived opposite me at no.3 and she never had no labour. She
used to be cleaning her windows. She used to be on the
chair, cleaning her windows, and a boy come up to my door
and he says, 'Lady over there wants you'. And I looked out
and I'd say, 'All right lad'. You know, take me apron and
that and go over. And perhaps I'd just have the chance,
maybe, to get her sitting on the chair. Soon as she sat on
the chair, the baby come – didn't want it in there no more!

It's surprising though. Some people don't have labour. It's very rare. They have the bearing down but they don't have no other pains. She had two little girls, both come like that. Mysterious, isn't it? But you could go home sooner! It's good for the midwife as well as the woman!

The midwives we spoke to were all much more rigid than Mrs G. in their attitude towards the position in which women gave birth. While principles of what is now called 'active birth'[6] were applied in the first stage of labour, it seems that all midwives insisted that the woman got onto the bed in second stage. They were very directive about the position for the birth in order to carry out what they saw as a most vital midwifery skill – 'the protection of the perineum':

> We delivered them in the left lateral [on the left side]. You could support the patient's leg around your neck, you see – you sort of made your hands tight together, flexed the head and let it crawl out slowly, very , very slowly. You had the odd skin nicks but you didn't have a lot of what I would call torn perineums. (*Elizabeth C.*)

Although episiotomies (cutting the women's vagina to speed up the delivery of the baby and prevent natural tearing) are done less routinely at present than ten years ago, they are still common in most hospitals. This horrifies midwives like Elsie B.:

> I don't think they're doing so many now, but there used to be all these episiotomies! And the whole thing that we trained for was to protect the perineum, not to split it. And the people used not to have half the trouble afterwards that they do today. Once you do one of those awful things, you've had it for next time. And you know, you used not to get the trouble with the babies that they say you'll get if you don't do them. I think they're going to die out probably.

The baby at birth

> I used to just hang it up by the feet. And funny, it nearly always used to start yelling...

Midwives working without oxygen and resuscitation equipment would resort to all sorts of methods to get the baby breathing. Methods ranged from the standard practice of holding the baby by its feet to that of dunking it in an ice-cold water butt to shock it into existence. Margaret A. describes the methods she used:

> On occasions, I've had to use mouth-to-mouth resuscitation, not very often. But with a baby that won't breathe you take hold of its feet and pat the bottoms of its feet – or another thing, too – blow in the centre of their stomachs like that – oooh – right in the centre of their tummies. And you often hear them go, 'aaaagh' [breathes in] if you do that. Not a wide blow, a thin blow right in the middle of their tummies. And I did have a doctor who would light a cigarette and blow cigarette smoke in the baby's face – oh, but I don't like that. It probably irritates the mucous membrane. I wouldn't do it – but then I don't smoke!

In the days when rupturing the membranes was not done routinely, occasionally babies were born 'in the caul', as Esther S. describes:

> Where the membranes haven't ruptured, you've got to watch 'cause if it does happen like that (a quick delivery – it could happen, you see), of course you have to whip it off. I had just a few. I got one off – oh, it was such a feature in the home. It was laid out and they tried to dry it. It was going to be given to someone in the family who was a sailor so that he would never drown. He'd go to sea and he'd be safe! In the war, every seaman tried to get one. If you carried one in your wallet, you wouldn't drown! Only a yarn, of course! But it was quite fun that!

The delivery of the placenta

> After they'd seen to the baby, the nurse always said, 'Now, go steady and just bear down gradually'. After you'd relaxed a little while after having your baby, then you'd bear down, they'd get the placenta out, and then they'd clamp it. My afterbirth was always brought out before the cord was cut.

The fact that Sissy S. remembers accurate details about the final part of labour [the third stage] is indicative of an age where women saw expelling the placenta as being part of the process of giving birth. Today, as the baby is being born, most women are routinely given an injection of an oxytocic drug to make the uterus contract strongly. Their attendant then pulls out the placenta and membranes for them, having clamped and cut the cord. Therefore, for most woman the process of giving birth stops at the baby; the rest is accomplished by the midwife.

Controversy over the effects of intervening in the third stage of labour continues. Many midwives complain that they have no experience of physiological (natural) third stage. It is, therefore, all the more interesting to hear the following midwives talk about what they did in the third stage of labour. Much of what they recommend is to be found in current literature on the subject:[7]

> *Mary W.*: I was taught to expel the placenta by fundal pressure [pressing on the top of the uterus], but as I got older, I used to leave the mother to do her own third stage, and I found it very much easier. You get them relaxed and then the third stage is never very much trouble – unless, of course, there's bleeding, and then you'd use ergometrine. At first, we used liquid ergot and then later on we could give the injection. Retained placentas were very rare. I can't think of more than a dozen times in 2,002 births, and then very few of those had to go into hospital for manual removal. That was very rare. We clamped and cut the cord after it stopped pulsating. We were taught that a certain amount of useful blood was given to the baby until the cord stops pulsating, so I always kept it that way.
>
> *Nellie H.*: Well, we just waited for it unless they were bleeding badly. We just went on waiting and then, well, we just used to catch it when it came out. It wasn't any bother. We'd encourage the mother, saying, 'Push with each pain, dear', but it didn't seem to cause any bother at all. Some took longer than others. If she was tight with it or got all excited, then it was sometimes a bit longer because she wasn't co-operating properly, but if the mother listened and did what she was told, it usually came out quite quickly – usually in five or ten minutes, but sometimes longer, often an hour. You'd transfer if it hadn't come after, say, twelve hours or so. You'd put it in a pail and check it over and then the husband would burn it down the garden.
>
> *Esther S.*: You just waited – you just kept your hand there to control and then when you found that the placenta was free, you just – down and out and that was it. I found that more midwives and doctors in the G.P. unit had retained placentas than ever I did – because they gave Syntometrine and then you've got to get it out quick before it's trapped. I don't like that at all. It's such a different way of delivering

– and the speed you lot have to work at! No, I like my own
old way. Usually, you had the placenta by 20 minutes – a
little 'show' and then you thought, 'Ah, that means its
separating – good!'

We used to feed the roses with the placenta – lovely! Now
they take them away, don't they? Or we'd burn them in
the house. Sometimes we used to whip one out – a nice
healthy one and take it home and dig it in the garden –
ever so good for roses. But normally you wrapped it up in
newspaper. It was quite a feature in the home. They all had
coal fires you see – it was lovely for delivery, a little coal
fire – and we used to put them on there and then we used
to count how many times it popped. If it pops three times,
there's another baby will come! I had one cord that was
47 inches long and once the cord was wrapped round
the baby's neck five times – it was a complete collar. How
it survived I'll never know.

Handywoman Mrs G., had obviously received some instruction
about the third stage of labour from her mother, who was a
trained midwife practising at the turn of the century:

When the baby's out, you wipe its eyes and mouth, put your
finger in its mouth and with the cotton wool bring out all
the blood – otherwise it would have swallowed the blood
and choked. And then, before the afterbirth comes, you
have to time the blood pressure; you hold the cord and then
you have to count the beats. It's OK. So then you hold it
about four inches away from the baby and then you double
it like this and then hold it like that for a while. You'd
double it over and then tie it with flax in those days. But
you don't cut in that loop, you cut the other end of the cord.
Yes, that's before the afterbirth comes out.

What happened if the afterbirth didn't come? Well, it had
to come, didn't it. And if it didn't, you had to force it. Well,
you'd press on the stomach, say, 'Come on, go to the
toilet, onto the can – not the front, the back'. And in those
days you used to fix towels to the bottom of the bed, you
know, twisted towels. And you used to put the towel in her
hands and say, 'Now hold that, and when you feel a pain,
think your horse is going to have a jump and PULL!' And
that helps you see, it forces it down and there you are.

When you get the afterbirth you have to see there's
none broken off. If there's a bit broken off, then you have

to find it in the blood as it comes out, otherwise it mortifies and then there's trouble. That's it, that's how it goes on. It's a lot of rigmarole really, isn't it. All these things. I think it's very interesting work.

Coping with emergencies

Elsie B., who spent all her working life in rural Devon starting in the 1930s, describes the isolation that many of the midwives had to cope with while carrying out their professional duties:

> When you were in some of the country areas you often had 30 miles to go to a consultant hospital. I think you had to know what you were doing as much then as you have to today – maybe more so? We only had the odd case of haemorrhage and we did have ergometrine, which was a great thing. One case in particular I remember and that was a very severe haemorrhage. We hadn't a doctor booked and the woman made a mistake. You see, it was difficult to get case histories always. Well, half of these things you didn't think about... What she failed to tell us was that, if ever she cut herself, she bled badly. You see, they didn't realise things and you had no idea... Well, I was five miles from a doctor and another two miles from a telephone. Anyway the husband was very good and he went to the telephone, but unfortunately you had to rouse the post-office people. And they didn't want to get up! The doctor was mad about that. You had to do compression to stop the bleeding. The woman was all right afterwards and the baby was all right. It took quite a number of weeks for her to pull up. That was the worst one I did, the only one really, and I must say I was very lucky. We didn't have much trouble with the babies either.

Mollie T. describes methods of dealing with haemorrhage that were being used in south-east London in the late 1940s:

> In my first period of training we used to give retention enemas of sweet coffee in cases of haemorrhage and shock [an alternative to intravenous re-hydration given by the rectum]. There was still a reluctance to give blood due to many more reactions with inadequate cross-matching, so we always had these large Winchesters [glass jars] of what looked like black treacle. We gave a retention enema of about six ounces of this very viscid material. The sugar and

caffeine were easily absorbed [through the blood supply in the rectum]... I never saw it kill anyone and they all got better with it!

The thing that worried me as a pupil midwife was that at that time, it was absolutely forbidden to give an oxytocic [a drug to make the uterus contract firmly] with the placenta in situ, and I don't know how you were supposed to stop any bleeding because you weren't supposed to interfere with the uterus when the placenta was inside either. I thought the only thing left to do was to pray on those occasions! [laughs]

The other thing we used a lot up till late 1950 was intravenous acacia gum – a tacky, viscid solution – and it was prepared under protest and with great difficulty by the pharmacy. It was instead of plasma, and it was always available. Unlike plasma, it didn't go off and was very stable. It was the choice of a particular group of consultant obstetricians. Acacia gum certainly saved some lives. The idea was that if the district midwife called a doctor, somebody who took the call at the hospital would get the doctor on his bicycle with appropriate bags, and the morphia from the drugs cupboard, and a bottle of acacia gum solution in his pocket because that would keep the vein or circulating system from collapsing – the viscosity of it, I mean. So that would keep things going until the flying squads [emergency units that came out from the hospital with staff and equipment to help the midwife in dealing with an emergency at home] got there. The flying squads sometimes were heavily in demand with so many more home confinements.

In urban areas where there were medical training schools, the midwife who called out a doctor in an emergency could not guarantee that the doctor would have any more expertise than she had. Mollie T. describes the procedure for calling the doctor in an emergency and her anxieties about the reliability of such a system of back-up:

In relation to calling for medical aid, I have looked out an excerpt from an old medical journal (1926), and here's a poem in 'dog Latin' which translates:

'The Clerks – that was the medical students – were refreshing themselves with wine when a messenger came running quickly from the house. He said, "There's a case of a mother labouring". The man came from City Road with a red drum.'

Well, that was a little red token that was given to patients when they booked, to send in an emergency, and the midwife would send it if she wanted a doctor. You see, many of them – the midwives – didn't read or write, and the husband was often drunk, but you could get him staggering along with a token, even if you couldn't get him doing much else! The discs were originally wooden and later on, the ones I saw were Bakelite.

It was definitely an anxiety for me as a pupil that I couldn't believe that if I sent for the doctor I would get the help I needed. One of the consultants told me that as a medical student he was sent out to look after a woman in tenements in Liverpool Road, and he'd never seen a delivery at all, though he'd had a few lectures. He sat beside the women – he was a nice chap – he was holding her hand and reading his textbook in the other and he got to the part about a full bladder holding up proceedings and she seemed to be making heavy weather of it, so he passed a catheter and the baby shot out!

So you see, it was no better training for doctors than it was for midwives. In fact, it was worse for the doctors because it was fairly common around the time I was a pupil for a midwife to be much more aware of the procedures, like how to put forceps on the head. She might well show the doctor how to do that and then show him how to carry out the traction, and she was probably skilled in breech delivery.

I remember I was in a situation in hospital where a houseman was the only doctor available for a breech delivery – all the nobs were in theatre – and I would perhaps have overruled him and done it myself, except that he was a nice fellow. He had got to start some time, so I talked him through by teaching the pupils, saying, 'In a moment you'll see the doctor do so and so...' We proceeded very nicely through this because he was a calm, sensible, competent fellow.

Five years ago, I met up with him somewhere and he said, 'There's one thing I remember was having to do a breech delivery and I really didn't know anything about it, and I don't know what I would have done if you hadn't taught the students'. I didn't have the heart to say, 'That's why I did it'. But he was still just as nice as ever...

Midwives are trained to deal with emergencies, and there will always be the rare, life-threatening situations where they find themselves coping alone. Such experiences are never forgotten, as Nellie H. explains:

> I will never forget this one night. This girl was bleeding badly [immediately after the birth] and I'd sent for the doctor, but he hadn't arrived because he was with another case. I could see that if I didn't do something she was going to bleed to death [the placenta had partially separated and needed to be removed so that the uterus could clamp down on the blood vessels and seal them off]. So I just scrubbed up, put on some gloves and peeled the placenta out. I mean I know you're not supposed to do that, but she'd have died. The doctor was ever so complimentary, but I was scared stiff. When he arrived, he said to the woman who was there, 'Take nurse down and make her a strong cup of tea'. I was hanging over the balcony, absolutely flabbergasted by what I'd done! Ah well, at least I know I've saved one life!

Although a breech birth at home would be considered an emergency nowadays, in pre-NHS days, such births were considered normal. All the midwives who spoke with us were skilled at delivering breech babies at home. Mary W. explains:

> When I was training pupils in the 1950s and 1960s, one thing that amazed me was that these pupils were never taught how to conduct a breech delivery. I mean, you know, how ever careful you are, how ever good your antenatal care, a breech can be missed. You can be landed with a breech delivery at home. These girls hadn't a clue about a breech delivery. It's a skill that you acquire. When I trained, you were taught that a breech was just another presentation and you had to cope with it. It's a shame these skills are being lost.

Edie B.'s face lit up with delight on hearing that one of the authors had been a 'breech baby', and her hands followed an imaginary and familiar set of manoeuvres as she enthused about breech births:

Oh, I used to *love* delivering breeches. The breech births are easy. Beautiful! You normally got the buttocks presenting and coming down so you just put your hand up and release a little foot and bring it out, a little twist and a little twist and release the other arm. Give it a little push and out the head comes. *Beautiful! Perfect!* And we never used to have problems with them.

The postnatal period

After she had the baby, she wasn't allowed up for ten days and then she just put her feet out of the bed and dangled them. They lay flat for three days in hospital. We had a lot of 'white legs', you know, DVTs [obstruction in the veins of the legs by the formation of blood clots]. They died from it you know.

Here, midwife Mary W. describes the risks of the well-meaning but rigid policy adopted in the first half of the century – that of 'confining' women to bed for at least ten days. Ivy D. explained why she obeyed this rule:

They said if I didn't all my insides would drop out and I didn't want that, did I. Still, it gave you a rest, but when the ten days were up you were expected to get up and do everything. His food had to be on the table, everything back to normal.

The ten-day ruling meant a lot of extra work for the district midwife. Mary W. remembers:

We went in to swab them and to make the beds. Occasionally the mother would make the bed, but it was very rare. 'Nurse' was given 30 shillings to do this, she was getting paid! So yes, you swabbed them and then bathed the baby – that was for eight days – and on the tenth day you showed them how to bathe the baby and they could then do it themselves. But it was very hard work.

Caring for mother and baby in the immediate postnatal period was hard work indeed if midwives followed instructions such as those laid down in Alice Gregory's 1923 midwifery textbook:

In order to refresh memories, I add the proper ritual for an ordinary morning visit – with no complications:
1. Ask at door for kettle and slop pail.

2. Remove cloak and leave outside bedroom. Roll up sleeves to elbow.

3. Open your bag, and the drawer holding napkins.

4. Wash, domestically, in cold water.

5. Give thermometer, open wool bag, mix lotions, perchloride of mercury, 1 – 1,000-quart basin, lysol in a second bowl, place these on a chair near bed.

6. Take and record pulse, temperature, respirations, look at tongue, ask if bowels are open, and other questions.

7. Remove binder, fold it up and place on pillow.

8. Put patient on clean chamber, with pillow in small of back.

9. Place paper receiver under bed.

10. Scrub and disinfect (two minutes' scrub, rinse, one minute soak, longer for lacerations, time by clock).

11. Take wool from wool bag and close its mouth, put swabs in lysol, one or two in perchloride of mercury solution and some in mouth of bag for breasts.

12. Soak hands again, push back clothes with elbow, lather with soap and lysol and stream down with that, then with perchloride of mercury. (The opening should be cleansed first and then covered with thin wet swab while the rest is lathered. Do not separate labia unless there are abrasions. These must be irrigated with either boracic or saline solution, or sterilised water, from sterilised bottle).

13. Remove chamber with left hand, and tilt patient onto side with right elbow.

14. Finish bathing from back, apply napkin, turn patient on back.

15. Scrub hands again, empty and refill basin.

16. Remove sheets and nightgown.

17. Soak hands in perchloride of mercury.

18. Wash and dry breasts with clean wool – cover with clean napkin.

19. Wash in the ordinary way face, hands, arms, abdomen and back.

20. Roll in binder, replace nightgown.

21. Rub uterus for five minutes, measure, adjust binder.

22. Do hair, cut nails if necessary.

23. Make bed, transferring patient to other side if possible.

24. Pin mother's flannel and towel together.

25. Scrub and soak hands one minute.

26. Wash infant before fire, beginning with eyes and mouth. Powder must be warm (not hot) and dry.

27. Empty basin, wash soap dish, leave nail brush in empty lotion bowl.

28. Rinse out chamber with perchloride of mercury, using breast swabs.

29. Empty pail, remove soiled linen, burn swabs.

30. Give full instructions to last till next visit. (All linen should be folded neatly and placed together as soon as it is taken from bed of patient. Feet should be washed once a week, and toe nails cut. The visit should last about one hour to one hour and a quarter, unless breasts have to be relieved or a catheter passed, when it maybe longer.)[8]

Such a routine is a far cry from the work of contemporary community midwives, who may have to fit in as many as sixteen postnatal visits in a day. Today, though, women are not 'confined' to bed and are encouraged to be active immediately following birth in order to avoid the risk of deep-vein thrombosis.

Midwives undoubtedly meant well in their strict efforts to keep women resting in bed for ten days, and were only too aware of how hard women had to work once they got up. Alice Gregory's book again:

> The working man is extremely uncomfortable as to his meals and home life generally, as long as his wife is in bed, and will hail with joy the moment she gets up as the moment when he may hope to return to his average level of comfort. Nothing but the most authoritative order from the doctor or midwife will ever keep the working woman in bed after the tenth day, and if she is once up she has got to work hard – don't make any mistake about that, whatever lies are told to the contrary.[9]

Edie B. described the rigid routine imposed on women 'confined' in hospitals. In the present day, when most women in Britain leave hospital within a couple of days of giving birth, it is worth noting that a similar routine was still in operation when one of the authors had her first baby in hospital in the late 1960s:

> They weren't allowed up for ten days. For the first two days after delivery, they were not allowed more than a cup of Bovril and toast for lunch – oh dear, the restriction on food! I've always thought they needed a jolly good feed after all that hard work. But no, 'Bovril and toast!' I can't think what the reasoning was, unless they'd got their anatomy mixed up and thought that the baby came from the stomach

and the stomach needed a rest! [laughter] Breakfast, of course, was porridge. On the third day, they were allowed fish for two days. Until the fourth day, they were not allowed a proper meal. I think many of the fathers used to bring in pork pies and things at night, you know! On the fifth day, they were given a blanket bath – that was blanket bath day. On the ninth day, they could get up. On the eleventh or twelfth days, they could go to the toilet. On the thirteenth day, they were allowed to see their babies bathed. We taught them how to bath baby. On the fourteenth day, they went home. The babies were in the nursery at night and by the mothers during the day. And they were fed rigidly every four hours, whether they cried or not.

On the whole, midwives actively discouraged the practice of babies being in the bed with the mother. However, Katherine L. described a situation where commonsense overrode the prevailing 'rules':

Did the babies sleep in the mother's bed? – No, well, I hope not, though I'm not going to say never because on one or two occasions when the weather was very cold and the babies were suckling like the twins we had at the top of Windmill Hill – a very, very cold flat. They'd done their level best to get it warm, but those twins suffered from – in the old days it wasn't called hypothermia, it was called lardacious disease. Now there's a nice word for you – 'lardacious'. Because the babies looked like lard, they said. Never seen it in print, but I hear the doctor call it that. So anyway, we put them in the mother's bed to keep them warm – but on the whole it didn't happen.

Josephine M. thought that the practice of keeping babies in the bed was prevalent in the East End of London for good reasons:

They didn't put them in cots. Put them in the bed. They sleep all night if it's in the bed. It won't sleep if it's out of the bed, will it?

Several of the midwives told us that they do not remember babies dying from cot death. Handywoman Mrs G had a theory that has since been validated by research:

And another thing, these days I believe they lay the babies down on their face. Well, I don't believe in that. We never put our babies down on their face, always on the back so that they can get the air. No wonder there are so many cot deaths, poor little mites! 'Cause I mean what sense has he got to turn himself over, he's not that clever. We never had no cot deaths.

Breast-feeding

Mrs G.'s wisdom did not extend to breast-feeding, however, and she had no belief in its potential benefits:

> I never fed any of mine. Never had a drop. I fed them on Robinson's Patent Groats [cereal]. You made it up thin and then they drank it through the bottle. Finest thing to feed a baby on, I think.

Josephine M. advocated breast-feeding according to the strict routine recommended by all the literature of the day:

> Demand feeding? Oh no, no – by the clock. Oh no, this demand feeding is a lot of nonsense! You take, for instance, yourself [to Billie]. You've got a baby, you've got a kitchen, you've got a husband. You've got a dinner to get, you've got your washing to do, your ironing – how can you drop tools every five minutes and feed a baby? It's a lot of nonsense.

Breast-feeding at predetermined intervals was by no means advocated by all midwives. Most midwives working in the community admitted that they knew that the officially advocated four-hourly, carefully timed feeding routine – still advocated until the early 1980s – was counter-productive. Take, for instance, Mary W., working in Yorkshire:

> I never really insisted on clock feeding because you were fighting a losing battle anyway. If you can get a baby going by the clock, all well and good, but if you can't, you can't. Some babies you can. We used to get a lot of breast abscesses. You can't imagine what it was like because you had to poultice them and then the doctor had to open it and drain out the pus – and then subsequent babies it was difficult and very often they couldn't feed.
>
> I think it was so common because they used to get cracked nipples. And I'll tell you what else – if they used to get engorged breasts women would say, 'Let your husband suck it out'. Well, you only had to have dental

cavities and your infection was there to start with. We used Vaseline or lanolin on cracked nipples, but often they'd stop breast-feeding on it.

Katherine L. and her sister, Margaret A., remembered advising women to use lead nipple shields to cope with cracked nipples:

> For cracked nipples we used these lead shields – that was something from Charlotte's [Queen Charlotte's Hospital], wasn't it? It was marvellous, but mind you, it became unpopular because of the lead. It's a bit hazardous but it clears them up ever so quickly. A piece of soft lead in the shape of the nipple sort of gouged out of it, which you put over a crack – and it was incredible how they would heal underneath it. But you had to be extremely careful and you daren't give them to a mother that wasn't sensible. You had to make sure she was going to clean herself to get rid of the lead, clean herself beforehand. Otherwise, baby would be sucking lead. They wore them in between feeds. It was the lead that cured the cracks, like a lead lotion, and it also kept the clothes from rubbing on the nipple.
>
> If you weren't going to breast-feed – and it's all a question of fashion – then they'd give them stilboestrol [synthetic oestrogen] to dry up the milk, and that would make them go all smelly and nasty. They don't give that anymore, do they, because of the risks of cancer. It was ever so common in our day.

Mary W. mentioned the decline in breast-feeding due to women's need to work, as described in Chapter 9:

> A lot of these women went out to work, and then the mothers looked after the babies and it was so much easier for the mothers to use a bottle. Also, the doctors weren't very good about insisting on breast-feeding and they'd say, 'Oh, well, put it on the bottle'. They'd start off breast-feeding, and then you'd find they'd given up by the end of the month. Dried milk was on by then, but a lot used cow's milk. I tell you what a lot of them used to use and couldn't get them away from it – Nestle's condensed milk.

Powdered milk companies were beginning to advocate artificial feeding for babies in the 1920s. Advertisements extolled the virtues of drinks such as 'Glaxo' for both mother and baby. *Nursing Notes*, the midwives' journal of that day, had the following advertisement:

Find in Glaxo a most valuable aid for, taken regularly two or three times a day by the mother herself (both before and after the birth of her baby), Glaxo not only maintains the mother's own strength without taxing her digestion, but also enriches and increases the flow of breast milk. This is because milk makes milk, and Glaxo is the nourishing solids of the finest milk and cream made germ-free and comfortably digestible by the Glaxo Process.

Should the breast milk fail from any cause, or not nourish Baby satisfactorily, Glaxo can be given to Baby in turn with the breast or as the sole food from birth, for it contains everything to nourish Baby and nothing to cause him harm.[10]

While today's mothers are not encouraged to drink the same formula milk as their babies, the promotion tactics of the formula milk companies will be familiar to all readers of the present-day equivalent to *Nursing Notes – The Midwives Chronicle*.

Postnatal depression

There wasn't time! They hadn't time to be postnatally depressed, love!

Mary W. countered the popular notion that women did not have the time for postnatal depression. When the subject was broached, she gave us two examples:

I have seen some. This girl, ever such a nice girl she was, she had delusions – thought the baby wasn't being looked after properly and that the woman who was looking after her wasn't doing her work properly. And I thought – 'This girl is curious'. So I said to the doctor, 'I want to watch this girl. I think she ought to go into hospital somewhere. I think she's going in for puerperal insanity'. He got somebody out and they certified this girl, which I didn't think ought to have been done. She went into a mental hospital – and she's never been out since. This must have been 40-odd years ago or more [the 1940s]. Of course, nowadays they would probably have given her shock treatment.

I had another one. She had, not a puerperal depression, but a condition anyway. She was lethargic, you know, and she'd previously had a baby that she'd gone queer with. So this same doctor got this psychiatrist out (they had a

> business, you know) and he gave her shock treatment at
> home. And she's been all right since. So I said to the doctor
> afterwards, 'Have you said anything to her husband about
> not having any more children?' He said, 'No, why should
> I?' And I said, 'Well, I think you ought. This woman ought
> not to have more children. If she's had two puerperal
> insanities she oughtn't to have any more children'. But it
> hadn't occurred to the man himself.
>
> Actually we have had puerperal depressions and so forth
> from time to time, but it was not very common. As I say,
> they just didn't have time to be depressed in the old days.

It is likely that, as today, a lot of postnatal depression went
unrecognised. Severe cases were hospitalised but, unlike today,
many women were never discharged from psychiatric care.

The art of midwifery

Whatever we may think about the attitudes of some of the
midwives quoted in regard to their practice, there can be no
doubt that they were true practitioners in their own right, and that
they understood the tried and tested midwifery art of patience.
What also comes across is the industrious nature with which
they approached their work.

Subsequent to the authors' own midwifery training, there have
been many shifts in practice. For example, there is a move afoot
towards creating a more 'woman-led' approach with less intervention in what, for most women, is a normal, healthy process.
Already, the prophecy of Edie B., interviewed seven years ago, is
coming true:

> I've seen lots of changes. Sometimes I wonder if it's all
> carried too far. I've got an awful feeling that you're going
> to drop some of it later – maybe I shall never see it – but I
> think it's all gone a bit too far.

Whatever changes in midwifery practice and ideology have
taken place over the years, there are basic attributes acknowledged
as important by midwives of all generations. When asked about
the important qualities for a midwife to possess, the following were
some typical responses:

> Understanding. It's no good just learning theory. Practice
> is the thing... (*Edie B.*)

I think you need some commonsense. You need to find a way to get on with people and not be too bossy. And you've got to be able to instil confidence. (*Elsie B.*)

Kindness for one thing. You have to be in sympathy with the woman. And patience and love of the job. (*Elsie* K.)

You've got to be capable of working on your own in adverse circumstances, make up your own mind, and having done it, carry it through. And if you've made a mistake, you can't afford to put your head in the sand and say, 'How awful!' You have to learn by your mistakes. This I think is what it is all about. (*Mollie T.*)

Practical, down-to-earth knowledge is important, but it's having the right attitude that's so important, too. You have to be their friend. If you can befriend a mother and get her on a level with you, there's an understanding and you're both far better off. I think the midwife in her own mind should remember that the mother is important to her. She, the midwife, is not the most important person. She isn't. The mother is the most important person. (*Esther S.*)

Elsie was always cheerful. She was chirpy, very sociable but she wasn't rowdy. She wasn't loud. She was thoughtful and she looked after the women. There was never a cross word. (*Mary T.*)

I think the most important thing is liking the mother. You know, when somebody comes and sits on your couch and says they're going to have a baby, you think, 'Oh, you're going to see something come into the world from this mother'. And you get extremely fond of your patients – well, some of them you don't – but mostly you have a feeling for them, don't you? Even the tarts of the village. Oh, we've had some marvellous tarts, haven't we, Marg?! (*Katherine L.*)

Patience, tact and sympathy – the whole charter if you're going to do it satisfactorily. (*Elizabeth C.*)

References

1. Campbell, R. and Macfarlane, A., *Where to be Born – The Debate and the Evidence*, National Perinatal Epidemiology Unit, Oxford, 1987, p.12.
2. *Central Midwives Board Rules 1934.*
3. Gregory, Alice (ed.), *The Midwife: Her Book*, Frowde & Hodder & Stoughton, London, 1923, p.25.

4. *ibid*, pp.22–24.
5. Odent, Michel, *Birth Reborn*, Souvenir Press, London, 1984.
6. Balaskas, Janet, *New Active Birth*, Thorsons, London, 1989.
7. Inch, Sally, *Birthrights – A Parent's Guide to Modern Childbirth*, Green Print, London, 1989, Chapter 7, pp.145–191.
8. Gregory, Alice (ed.), *op. cit*, pp.20–21.
9. *op. cit*, p.39.
10. *Nursing Notes*, November 1920.

Postscript: a tribute to the women in this book

I feel as tough as nails. I don't inwardly. Inwardly, I feel very, very sad, terribly sad. But outwardly, I always put on a show. It doesn't matter what might happen. Come what may, I always put on that show. Sometimes I feel like a clown wending my way through life, you've got to giggle and laugh – and inside it bleeds for such a lot of things. But then, once again, it's life, it's all happened – and crying now won't help. (*Edie M.*)

Having a baby with Nurse Walkerdine, I can't express it. It was marvellous, just marvellous. She was an angel through and through. If you needed bed clothes, that nurse found them. In them days, you often relied on neighbours if you never had nothing. And Nurse W. always found things for you. She'd say, 'We'll see if we can find you some bits'. (*Sissy S.*)

Recently, I've been thinking about how midwifery has developed over the years since the days of the handywoman. I think one always remembers the worst, and after that the best, and nothing in between. I can't think that people have changed at all over the years, perhaps slightly different proportions. I should think we've probably still got a very small quantity of 'Sairey Gamps', but undoubtedly the average is always tending upwards and I think that of the upper echelons of the elite there are some of those that are extraordinarily competent and some that are very academic. This hasn't changed a great deal, but that the academic lot wouldn't have been there in Dickens's time. We're talking about human beings, and they haven't changed. Even with good training, you always have the bossy midwife with the best intentions, and yet apparently totally unfeeling in everything she says and does. I suppose we'll always have that person, and you'll always have somebody trying to tone them down, too. You can try to influence them in training. You can try to counsel them out of midwifery, but the difficulty is, they'll very probably want to stay because it offers independence.

I don't know whether you go into midwifery because you're a bit of a square peg in a round hole or whether you get like it. Maybe it's a bit of both, but midwifery has always attracted individualists.

You learn a lot as an observer of midwifery. It sounds as though I'm painting a very negative picture – I suppose being a teacher of midwives as well, one is well aware of the need to change or correct something – but I think that over the considerable amount of years that I've been observing, the overall impression is that I'm surprised that midwives do so much and so well in such adverse circumstances. (*Mollie T.*)

Methodology: using oral history in midwifery research

Traditional textbook history rarely deals with the everyday, commonplace experiences of most people's lives. It focuses on events – often using interviews or diaries of government ministers or members of the royal family. What we do not read, however, is what went on behind the scenes: how ordinary people felt, what they wore or ate, or the details of everyday life. Most of all, women's experiences are absent, often because they were never recorded in the first place. Whole areas of women's history have been 'forgotten'.

It seemed to us, as practising midwives, that there has been a very particular gap in midwifery history. Some excellent historical overviews have been written, documenting the evolution of the midwifery profession (*see* Bibliography), but no-one appeared to have recorded the testimonies of women who worked as midwives in the first half of this century. This period is especially important since many changes in midwifery practice and legislation were occurring that were significant in the development of the profession.

Getting started

We decided to interview retired midwives and women who gave birth in the first half of this century, in order to try to piece together a more complete picture of the lives of childbearing women and those who attended them. The formation of the National Health Service (NHS) in 1948 brought dramatic changes, so this seemed a natural boundary for our research. We also decided to limit the interviews to people living in the British Isles.

Encouraged by our first interviews with retired midwives whom we knew, we decided, in 1985, to collect more testimonies and shape them into a book. We sent letters to the *Midwives Chronicle*, to midwives who attended the retired midwives' Christmas party at the Royal College of Midwives, and to the local papers asking for potential interviewees. We visited two day centres for the elderly and discussed our project with women there. The response was encouraging.

The interviews

With one exception – Ken W., whose vivid memories of his mother, a handywoman, form an important testimony – all of the interviews were with women. Each interview took place in the interviewee's home, apart from two which took place in the day centres. Before starting each interview, we agreed a length of time that it would last, bearing in mind that elderly people often tire easily and that we were guests in their homes.

We made sure that the interviewees understood that we would be using the material for publication and explained that we would use their first name plus the initial of their surname in any published text in order to preserve their anonymity. We asked if we could use a tape recorder during the interview to avoid the intrusion that can be caused by the constant use of a notebook. Although some people felt initially nervous about this, they expressed surprise, in retrospect, at how quickly they forgot its presence once the interview was underway.

We prepared a checklist of topics to cover, but as our confidence in interviewing developed, we referred to it less and less. We learned that asking open-ended questions and allowing silences resulted in far richer material. We also learned that sometimes you have to 'stop the flow' tactfully, for instance after ten minutes of monologue about variations on 'baby's layette'.

The midwives' testimony

Interviews with the midwives were often enhanced when a two-way process of discussion about midwifery practice was allowed to develop. Our contempory experience was often of interest to the older women, and memories would be triggered as we compared notes about the similarities as well as the changes that have occurred over the years.

Most midwives we interviewed had spent the whole of their working lives in the profession. They had a strong sense of professional identity and still read the *Midwives Chronicle* to keep themselves up to date. Usually, they were very enthusiastic and eager to reminisce, and it seemed as if the interview gave them a chance to relive their experiences and to re-establish their sense of self-worth.

We were amazed at the detail of the midwives' memories, and particularly at their ability to recite whole paragraphs of midwifery textbooks verbatim – details they had learned 60 years previously, repeated with the rigid conviction that had been expected of them all those years ago. This 'going by the rules' approach was disappointing, as we had approached the interviewing with a naive expectation that we would be uncovering a host of forgotten skills, a treasure chest of tips and ideas.

Our romantic expectations were to be dashed in other ways too. We were often shocked, for example, by the authoritarian manner of the midwives. Many implied that they would go into women's homes and lay down the law in order to 'educate' people. As one midwife put it:

> They had to be taught to be good mothers. Some of them were very foolish and irresponsible.

On the whole, the working-class midwives we interviewed appeared to have more empathy with the women they attended. They talked more openly and appeared to enjoy telling stories. We are aware that, therefore, a large part of the book is shaped around their testimony, and also that this class difference might have been due to the particular women who agreed to talk to us.

Transcribing and editing

> Transcribing is undoubtedly very time-consuming, as well as being a highly skilled task. It takes at least six hours, and for a recording with difficult speech or dialect up to twice as long, for each hour of recorded tape.[1]

The transcripts were written exactly as the women spoke, but we only included phonetic renderings of speech if these were relevant to an accurate conveyance of meaning. All 'umms' and 'ers' were originally retained in the transcripts. Later, they were mostly edited out, as were any repetitions, unless they were significant, for example, if they portrayed someone's embarrassment or sorrow.

Editing the transcripts presented us with dilemmas. How could we edit such lively, diverse reminiscences? So much of the material was riveting. There was a temptation to select humorous or shocking stories at the expense of those that were more mundane, but possibly more representative. And what were we to do with remarks that we found distasteful – for instance, racist statements? We were shocked to find some of these warm-hearted, older women holding racist prejudices. However, we realised that the prejudices themselves are all part and parcel of women's experiences, and that it is not for us to select out only the parts that were 'ideologically sound'.

Reflections on issues in oral history

At the beginning of this project, as we started looking for women to interview, there was a sense of urgency. It felt vital to record the reminiscences of an older generation of midwives before it was too late to hear their stories. With a good deal of enthusiasm, we set off armed with tape recorders and notebooks (and Billie's three-month-old baby) to record the forgotten voices of the past and to rewrite history using the words of women themselves.

Several interviews later, we stopped, feeling confused and anxious. We were going into people's homes, and by probing and asking questions, we were stirring up buried memories and evoking feelings that had often been put aside. Sometimes we were the only people the women had confided in, and much of the material was of a very intimate nature – a potential difficulty for women from a less 'explicit' generation. After the interview, we would walk out of their lives, possibly leaving them feeling exposed and vulnerable.

As we questioned what we were doing, oral history did not seem to be the egalitarian process that we had originally envisaged. We realised that, as interviewers, we had considerable power and that we could control the information we were given. We could encourage certain memories and block others merely by the tone of our voices or our body language.

We began to question our own role and motivation in the situation. What were *we* getting out of it all? We needed to accept the amount of power we had as interviewers and editors of the material, instead of naively pretending that we were just listening ears and the means by which the stories were put down on paper. Were we just taking and not giving back? How much could we realistically expect to offer in terms of friendship or support to these women, many of whom appeared lonely? There are no easy answers to these questions, but we feel that it is important that anyone undertaking research of this nature develops an awareness of the issues involved and a sensitivity to the dynamics of the interviewing situation.

We learned that it was important to see oral history as a reflection of the woman's personal history, affected by her class, religion, culture and politics. Rarely were memories told against a larger political backdrop. As so often happens today, local people or organisations were blamed when it was actually government policies that were creating the problem. Occasionally however, there were glimpses of a wider historical context, as in this quote from midwife, Nellie H.:

> When there was the General Strike in 1926, I was training in Plaistow. The policeman used to come and look after us and escort us along the road. The policeman came because people went absolutely mad. I don't think anybody realises what it was like unless they were alive then. They were throwing eggs, tomatoes and all sorts of things all over the place. There used to be big vans, full of men, all gone crazy. Throwing things at you. So the police had to guard us to get us safely to the mothers' homes.

As we did more interviews, we became more aware of the particular difficulties presented in the women's language itself, especially when women spoke with strong regional accents. How often were we missing some vital clue or nuance in what was said? In Chapter 6, for instance, we describe the process of discovering that many women referred to abortions as 'miscarriages', and how initially this confused our analysis of what they were telling us about women's control of their fertility.

One of the problems of interpreting oral evidence is that people's memories are selective. The 'truth' for them may not tally with the historical 'facts'. The women we interviewed rarely complained about how bad things had been for them. They tended to recall only happy times, and would dismiss the bad memories with sweeping generalisations. For instance, Josephine M., a midwife working in the East End in the 1930s, says:

> When you'd go to a family they'd just have one room and one little bed. They might have a sheet or two – they were very, very poor but grateful. They might have a rug or two

on the bed and no blanket. And if they'd got a drunken bum
of a husband, which was very often the case, as long as he
got money for a drink that's all he cared. Life was really hard.
Coal fires and a gas lamp. But they were very happy.

References to the 'happy poor' cropped up time and time again,
and are hard to untangle. Perhaps memories of bad times have
been repressed because they are too painful. It also seemed that
women had an investment in holding onto the good things
there had been, so that they could talk about their lives with pride
and dignity. Most of the women we talked with combined
memories of poverty and hardship with those of happiness. There
were only a few who admitted that they had felt overwhelmingly
oppressed by their lives. Edie M. is one of these:

> Looking back, it was a horrible life. At that time, I used to
> accept it because we knew no other. You never knew
> carpets or fridges or heating... This old memory don't shut
> much out either. It goes over all the worst parts. Sometimes
> I have to block it out and think, 'Well, let's think of some
> nice things'. When I go to bed I have to. I think, 'Now, stop
> it Edie. Stop it Edie'. You've either got to take a second
> sleeping tablet, or you've got to block it out... You can't live
> with some things you've done...

Understandably, women's memories of the same situation
varied, even on factual points (e.g. the amount of dole money paid
out in the 1920s). Some midwives had difficulty remembering
when things happened and would describe situations that could
only have occurred in a later period than the one with which we
were concerned.

It also seemed that women sometimes told us what they
thought we would like to hear – things that they thought would
please us. This particularly happened when we interviewed the
midwives. They often answered questions as though they were
being 'tested' on their midwifery knowledge – hence the recitation
of whole chunks of midwifery textbook (referred to above).

It is possible that embarrassment on the part of the interviewees
may well have been a factor when we were researching the
chapter on women's knowledge about 'the facts of life'. Some
women may have felt too inhibited to discuss their sexuality
frankly, although we were often surprised and moved by the
intimate nature of some of the testimony.

So, how reliable *is* oral reminiscence? As discussed above, memories can be distorted because of poor or selective recall, a desire to please the interviewer or inhibition. At the end of the day, we have to settle for the fact that, in the words of oral historian Gilda O'Neill:

> Each version of a story has its own truth. And our myths, whether of the universal, numinous kind, or of the more prosaic family variety, are used by us to tell and retell truths in ways that mean we can make sense of our world.[2]

While acknowledging some of the limitations of oral history, we consider it to have radical potential. Without it, the memories of the women in this book would never have been passed on to more than a few relatives and friends. It is our hope that some of the testimonies that we have collected over the past seven years will inspire and educate readers as they have done for us.

References

1. Thompson, Paul, *The Voice of the Past – Oral History*, Oxford University Press, 1978, p.197.
2. O'Neill, Gilda, *Pull No More Bines*, The Women's Press, London, 1990, p.145.

Milestones in midwifery in 20th century, pre-NHS Britain

1902: First Midwives Act

Central Midwives Board set up for England and Wales with responsibility for: regulating, supervising and limiting practice; admission to and removal from the Roll; training; examinations; issuing and cancelling certificates; plenary board.

Local Supervising Authorities set up with responsibility for: supervising midwives; investigating malpractice; suspending midwives from practice in order to prevent the spread of infection; reporting malpractice and legal offences to the CMB; keeping a local list of midwives who notified their intention to practice annually; monitoring changes of address or deaths; ensuring midwives knew about the regulations and role of the CMB.

Admission to the Roll to be granted to:
1. those who already had a recognised midwifery qualification from the London Obstetrical Society (LOS) or certain lying-in hospitals;
2. women who could prove they were of good character who had already been in practice for at least one year – known as *bona fide* midwives;
3. those who could pass the CMB examination of competence following a three-month period of training.

1905

Publication of the First Roll of Midwives: 22,308 names – 9,787 had undertaken a course of midwifery training and 12,521 were *bona fide*.

From now on nobody could assume the title 'midwife' unless they had a certificate from the CMB.
LOS examination discontinued and first CMB examination.

1909

First antenatal clinic at Queen Charlotte's Hospital.

1910

Women who were not certified midwives were forbidden to attend women in childbirth 'habitually and for gain' except under the direction of a medical practitioner.

1911

National Insurance Act – workers to make a weekly compulsory payment entitling them to the services of a 'panel doctor' and to sickness and maternity benefits.

1915

Notification of birth after the 28th week now compulsory.

1916: First Scottish Midwives Act

Midwifery training period increased to six months (four months for those with nursing qualification).

1917

Report on the 'Physical Welfare of Mothers and Children England and Wales' by Dr Janet Campbell – the important role of the midwife highlighted; also her long hours and poor remuneration.

1918: Second Midwives Act

LSAs to be responsible for paying the doctors' fees in the first instance, but these fees still to be recovered from the patient if possible.
CMB given power to suspend midwives from practice. (Previously, they could only remove names from the Roll.)

Midwives to be compensated for loss of earnings if suspended from practice.

All forms and books that the midwife required to complete to be provided free, as well as postage for statutory notification forms.

MATERNAL AND CHILD WELFARE ACT: Local authorities encouraged to set up maternal and child welfare centres to include provision for antenatal clinics.

1919

A grant of £20 made available from the Treasury, payable to each pupil midwife who guaranteed to practise on qualification.

1923

Government report on 'The Training of Midwives' by Dr Janet Campbell highlighted the need for more trained midwives to reduce maternal mortality (static at four per 1,000 births between 1907 and 1922).

1926: Third Midwives Act

Uncertified women attending births were to satisfy a court that 'the attention was given in a case of sudden or urgent necessity'. Liable to a fine of up to £10.

Maternity homes to be legally required to register with the local LSA and be open for inspection.

Courses set up by the Midwives Institute for qualified midwives, followed by examination for the Midwife Teachers Certificate.

1927

CMB directive on advertising. 'All advertising to be deprecated and midwives ought to be satisfied with a plate on their doors, and cards'.

General Register Office's first tabulation of live births in England and Wales by place of delivery: 85 per cent of births taking place at home, 15 per cent in institutions.

1929

Government report on the working of the Midwives Act 1902–1926 saw the midwife as remaining the key provider of maternity care and highlighted areas of concern.

1930

The Ministry of Health authorised payment of fees to G.P.s for the routine examination of pregnant women who had engaged a midwife and who were not insured under the National Health Insurance Act.

1932

76 per cent of births occurred at home, 24 per cent in institutions.

1935

80 per cent of all pregnant women had some antenatal care.

1936 Midwives Act

LSAs in England and Wales charged with providing an adequate salaried midwifery service. This service to be subsidised by the government.
Midwives could choose to continue to work independently.
Compensation to be given to those who surrendered their certificates due to not wishing to become salaried or rejection by the LSAs.
Parturient women to pay the LSA for midwifery services, money to be collected by the midwives.
Midwives employed by LSAs now had 'off-duty', annual leave, pensions, provided equipment and uniforms plus financial security.
CMB to grant a Midwife Teacher's Diploma after examination.
Start of Statutory Refresher Courses for qualified midwives.
Residential Refresher Courses of seven days' duration at five-yearly intervals to be compulsory for all practising midwives.
Midwives returning to practice to undertake a course of instruction, the duration of which to be decided by the CMB.

Qualifications/requirements laid down for Supervisors of Midwives.

1937 Maternity Services (Scotland) Act

Similar reorganisation of maternity services in Scotland to that of the 1936 Midwives Act but all women having home births entitled to the services of a medical practitioner. 34.8 per cent of all births in England and Wales now took place in institutions.
Midwifery responsibility for postnatal care extended to 14 days.

1938

Midwifery training lengthened and divided into two parts, with an exam after each part: one year for State Registered Nurses, two years for non-nurses.

1939

Maternal mortality rate started to drop due to better distribution of wealth and benefits in the Second World War, improved housing and sanitation and overall rise in the standard of living. The introduction of sulphonomides, ergometrine, blood transfusions and emergency obstetric units also played a part. (By 1943, maternal mortality was half the 1935 rate, at 2.30 per 1,000 registered births: stillbirth rate 30 per 1,000.)
Emergency Powers (Defence)Act authorises LSAs to allow women whose names had been removed from the Roll to act as midwives in situations where there was a shortage. Midwifery designated as a form of National Service.

1941

Rushcliffe Committee set up to consider salaries and conditions of service for midwives.

1943

The Ministry of Labour and National Service highlighted the shortage of midwives and mounted a publicity campaign to attract more midwives.

The Employment of Women (Control of Engagement) Order required newly qualified midwives to practise for at least one year.

Rushcliffe Report identified midwifery as a 'distinct profession with its own traditions' and provided mechanisms for negotiations between midwives and their employing authorities. (Rushcliffe committee succeeded by Whitley Council in 1948.)

1944

55 per cent of babies born at home.

1946 NHS Act

The Beveridge Committee began to formulate proposals for social legislation and restructuring health services to deal with social and economic inequalities in Britain.

Shortage of midwives critical as birth rate reached its post-war peak. Midwifery training courses for State Enrolled Nurses instigated.

1947

CMB produced new-style Rule Book incorporating a Code of Practice.

1948 The National Health Service came into being

A comprehensive health service, free at the point of service, paid partly by contributions of those in employment, partly by local rates and partly from the General Exchequer funds.

The main source for this section is Towler, J. and Bramall, J., *Midwives in History and Society*, Croom Helm Ltd, Beckenham, Kent, 1986.

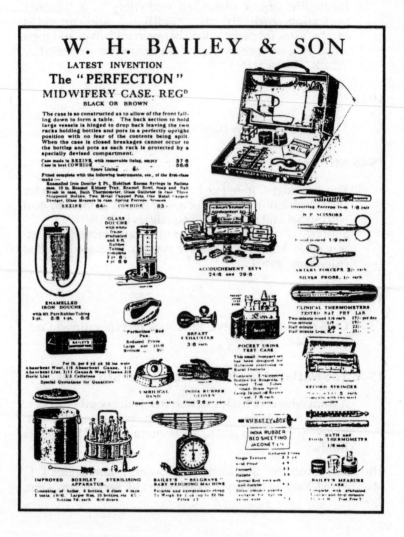

Advertisement for a midwifery case, 1925.

Glossary

***Bona fide* midwife** Midwife who registered under the 1902 Midwives Act. The Act allowed midwives who had been in practice for at least one year and who could produce written testimony of their good character to register under the Act and thereby practise midwifery legally. This was a stop-gap measure to cope with the shortage of trained midwives. The system of registering as a *bona fide* midwife was discontinued after 1905.

Breech Emergence of the baby's feet, knees or buttocks before the head in childbirth. A breech birth is recognised as being potentially more complicated and life-threatening for the baby.

Caul The amnion, or membrane enveloping the foetus and enclosing the liquor or 'waters'. Occasionally, it does not rupture and the baby is said to be born 'in the caul'. This is considered lucky in some folklore where the caul is endowed with properties for preventing drowning at sea.

Central Midwives Board (CMB) Regulatory body created under the 1902 Midwives Act. The Board designated and approved training institutions and teachers, set the syllabus and examinations for the CMB certificate, issued the certificate upon successful completion of training, formulated and codified rules by which the midwives' practice was defined and supervised and, in the event of suspected malpractice, procedures by which midwives would be investigated and disciplined.

Certified midwife A midwife who held a certificate from the CMB entitling her to practice.

Cervix Neck of the uterus

Cervical dilatation The opening of the cervix in the first stage of labour, caused by uterine contractions. When an internal examination is carried out through the vagina, the diameter of the opening is assessed. These days, it is recorded in centimetres.

Deep vein thrombosis (DVT) A blood clot in the veins of the legs, often caused by keeping women in bed too long after childbirth. The DVT can move through the bloodstream and block vital organs, such as the lungs, causing death.

Direct-entry training Midwifery training for those who do not have a nursing qualification.

Domiciliary At home. In the first half of this century, community or district midwives were often referred to as domiciliary midwives since they attended women in childbirth in their homes.

Ergometrine An oxytocic drug given to prevent or control haemorrhage in the third stage of labour by causing strong uterine contractions.

Grand multipara or **'grand multip'** A woman who has given birth to several children, usually at least four.

Handywoman Usually a working-class woman who attended women in childbirth but did not register as an official midwife. Known often as 'the woman you called for', most handywomen also laid out the dead. After 1910, handywomen could only practise under the direct supervision of a doctor, and after 1936, they were no longer allowed to practice at all. Some continued to work alongside the trained midwives, offering domestic duties in the postnatal period such as washing, cleaning, cooking and childcare.

Inspector of Midwives People appointed by the Local Supervising Authority to supervise and inspect midwives practising within their jurisdiction. They were also referred to as Supervisor of Midwives, the modern equivalent

Local Supervising Authority (LSA) County borough governments charged with ensuring that midwives were registered under the Midwives Act and that their practices conformed to the rules of the CMB.

Medical Officer of Health Public health physician appointed by the LSA to supervise and inspect midwives in their area.

Midwives Institute The organisation that sought to make midwifery into a profession for well-educated, middle-class women. Founded in 1881, it became the Royal College of Midwives in 1947.

Morbidity Damage, both mental and physical, in this case following childbirth.

Mortality rates

> **Maternal** The number of maternal deaths (due to pregnancy and childbearing) per 1,000 registered births.

> **Infant** The number of deaths of infants under one year per 1,000 registered live births.

Neonatal Infant deaths during the first four weeks of life per 1,000 registered live births.

Perinatal The number of stillbirths and neonatal deaths occurring during the first weeks of life per 1,000 total births.

Multiparous women or **'multips'** Women who have given birth to at least one viable baby.

Os The opening formed within the cervix.

Perineum The area around and between the vagina and the anus.

Placenta The afterbirth.

Placenta praevia A condition in which the placenta has implanted abnormally over the internal entrance to the cervix, blocking the way out for the baby and often causing severe haemorrhage.

Post-partum After giving birth.

Primipara or **'primip'** A woman having her first baby, or having given birth to one viable baby.

Puerperal fever/sepsis A condition associated with systemic bacterial infection and septicaemia that occurs following childbirth. It can be introduced by non-sterile hands or instruments inserted into the vagina and was once a major cause of maternal deaths.

Puerperium The six- to eight-week period following childbirth when the woman's uterus and other organs return to their pre-pregnant state (apart from her breasts if she is lactating).

Registered midwife Any midwife who was registered under the Midwives Act.

Stages of labour

> **First** The period from the onset of labour to complete dilatation of the cervix.

> **Second** The expulsive stage of labour, from full dilatation of the cervix to the complete birth of the baby.

> **Third** The period from the birth of the baby to the complete expulsion of the placenta and membranes.

Sulphonomides A group of drugs used to combat bacterial infections.

Trained midwife A midwife who had undergone formal training leading to a recognised examination, enabling her to register as a midwife.

Bibliography

Abel-Smith, B., *The Hospitals 1800–1948*, Heinemann, London, 1964.

Age Exchange. *What Did You Do in the War, Mum?: Women Recall Their Wartime Work*; *Fifty Years Ago, Memories of the 1930s: A Collage of Stories and Photographs of Day-to-day life around 1933*; *Of Whole Heart Cometh Hope: Centenary Memories of the Co-Operative Women's Guild*; *Can We Afford the Doctor?: Memories of Health Care*. All available from Age Exchange, Blackheath Village, London SE3.

Alison, Julia, 'Midwives Step Out of the Shadows' in *The Midwives Chronicle*, vol. 105, no. 1,254, July 1992.

Allan, P. and Jolley, M. (eds.), *Nursing, Midwifery and Health Visiting Since 1900*, Faber & Faber, London, 1982.

Arbuthnot Lane, Sir W. (ed.), *The Modern Woman's Home Doctor*, Odhams Press Ltd, London, 1930s.

Arms, Suzanne, *Immaculate Deception*, Bantam Books, New York, 1975.

Arney, W.R., *Power and the Profession of Obstetrics*, University of Chicago Press, 1982.

Balaskas, Janet, *New Active Birth*, Thorsons, London, 1989.

Beddoe, Deirdre, *Discovering Women's History*, Pandora Press, London, 1983.

Campbell, Rona and Macfarlane, Alison, *Where to be Born – The Debate and the Evidence*, National Perinatal Epidemiology Unit, Oxford, 1987.

Carter, Jenny and Duriez, Therese, *With Child – Birth through the Ages*, Mainstream Publishing Company (Edinburgh) Ltd, 1986.

Central Midwives Board Rules and *Central Midwives Board Annual Reports*, enquiries to United Kingdom Central Council for Nursing, Midwifery and Health Visiting, London.

Chamberlain, Mary, *Old Wives' Tales*, Virago Press, 1981.

Chamberlain, Mary, 'Life and Death', *Oral History – the Journal of the Oral History Society*, vol. 11, no. 1, spring 1983.

Chamberlain, Mary, *Growing Up in Lambeth*, Virago Press, 1989.

Cowell, Betty and Wainwright, David, *Behind the Blue Door – The History of the Royal College of Midwives 1881–1981*, Bailliere Tindall, London, 1981.

Davin, Anna, 'Imperialism and Motherhood', *History Workshop Journal*, spring, 1978.

Department of Health (Campbell, Janet), *Report on Public Health and Medical Subjects – No. 21 The Training of Midwives*, Whitehall, June 1923.

Department of Health, Maternal Mortality – *Report of Meeting Held at Central Hall, Westminster, on February 28th 1928*, published by The Maternal Mortality Committee, HMSO, London, 1928.

Department of Health, *Departmental Committee on Maternal Mortality and Morbidity 1930*, London, HMSO, 1930.

Department of Health, *House of Commons Health Committee Report on Maternity Services*, HMSO, London, 1992.

Dickens, Charles, *Martin Chuzzlewit*, Chapman & Hall, London, 1844.

Donnison, Jean, *Midwives and Medical Men*, Schocken Books, New York, 1977.

Ehrenreich, Barbara and English, Deirdre, *Witches Midwives and Nurses*, Writers and Readers Publishing Cooperative, London, 1973.

Fairbairn, John S., *A Textbook for Midwives*, 4th edition, Oxford University Press, 1924.

Fildes, Valerie, *Breasts, Bottles and Babies*, Edinburgh University Press, 1986.

Gittins, Diana, 'Married Life and Birth Control between the Wars', *Oral History – The Journal of the Oral History Society*, vol. 3, no. 2, autumn 1975.

Gregory, Alice (ed.), *The Midwife: Her Book*, Frowde & Hodder & Stoughton, London, 1923.

Hall, Ruth (ed.), *Dear Dr. Stopes – Sex in the 1920s*, Penguin, London, 1978.

Heagerty, Brooke, *Class, Gender and Professionalization: The Struggle for British Midwifery, 1900–1936*, Unpublished dissertation, 1990. Available in Royal College of Midwives' Library (reference only).

Holdsworth, Angela, *Out of the Dolls House*, BBC Books, London, 1988.

Inch, Sally, *Birthrights – A Parent's Guide to Modern Childbirth*, Green Print, London, 1989.

Jordan, Terry, *Agony Columns*, Optima, London, 1988.

Kenner, Charmian, *No Time For Women: Exploring Women's Health in the 1930s and Today*, Pandora Press, London, 1985.

Kitzinger, Sheila (ed.), *The Midwife Challenge*, Pandora Press, London, 1988.

Leavitt, Judith Walzer, *Brought to Bed: Child-Bearing in America 1750–1950*, Oxford University Press, 1986.

Lewis, Jane, *The Politics of Motherhood: Child and Maternal Welfare in England 1900–1939*, Croom Helm, London, 1980.

Lewis, Jane, *Women in England 1870–1950*, Wheatsheaf Books, Sussex, 1984.

Lewis, Jane (ed.), *Labour & Love – Women's Experience of Home and Family, 1850–1940*, Basil Blackwell, Oxford, 1986.

Liddiard, Mabel, *The Mothercraft Manual* (12th edition), Churchill, London, 1954.

Little, Bob, *'Go Seek Mrs. Dawson. She'll know what to do' – The Demise of the Working Class Nurse/Midwife in the Early Twentieth Century*. Unpublished Thesis, 1983. Sociology Dept., University of Essex.

Llewelyn Davies, Margaret (ed.), *Life as We Have Known it – by Co-operative Working Women*, re-printed by Virago, London, 1977. Published 1915 originally.

Llewelyn Davies, Margaret, *Maternity: Letters from Working Women*, Virago, London, 1978.

Messer, D., *Labour of Love*, New Horizon, Bognor Regis, 1981.

Morland, Egbert, *Alice and the Stork or the Rise in the Status of the Midwife as Exemplified in the Life of Alice Gregory 1867–1944*, Hodder & Stoughton, London, 1944.

Nursing Notes, 1890–1948, Journal of the Midwives Institute. Available (reference only) in the Royal College of Midwives' Library.

Oakley, Ann, 'Wisewoman and Medical Man: Changes in the Management of Childbirth' in *The Rights and Wrongs of Woman* (Juliet Mitchell and Ann Oakley, eds.), Penguin, London, 1976.

Oakley, Ann, *Women Confined: Towards a Sociology of Childbirth*, Schocken Books, New York, 1980.

Oakley, Ann, *The Captured Womb*, Basil Blackwell, Oxford, 1984.

Odent, Michel, *Birth Reborn*, Souvenir Press, London, 1984.

O'Neill, Gilda, *Pull No More Bines – an Oral History of East London Women Hop Pickers*, The Women's Press, London, 1990.

Porter, Marilyn, *Home, Work and Class Consciousness*, Manchester University Press, 1983.

Radcliffe, Walter, *Milestones in Midwifery*, John Wright & Sons, Bristol, 1967.

Reeves, Maud Pember, *Around About a Pound a Week*, Bell & Sons, Ltd., London, 1913. Re-printed by Virago, London, 1979.

Richardson, Ruth, in 'Laying Out and Lying In', *Association of Radical Midwives Newsletter*, July 1982.

Roberts, Elizabeth, *A Woman's Place – An Oral History of Working-class Women 1890–1940*, Basil Blackwell, Oxford, 1984.

Robertson, William H., *An Illustrated History of Contraception*, The Parthenon Publishing Group, Carnforth, Lancs, 1990.

Spring Rice, Margery, *Working Class Wives, Their Health and Conditions*, Penguin Books, London, 1939. Re-printed by Virago, London, 1981.

Stopes, Marie, *Married Love*, G.P. Putnam & Sons, London, 1918.

Tew, Marjorie, *Safer Childbirth: A Critical History of Maternity Care*, Chapman & Hall, London, 1990.

Thompson, Flora, Lark Rise to Candleford, Penguin Books Ltd., Harmondsworth, UK, 1978.

Thompson, Paul, *The Voice of the Past: Oral History*, Oxford University Press, 1984.

Thomson, Mary, *Stork's Nest*, unpublished autobiography describing midwifery training in the 1930s in Glasgow.

Thunhurst, Colin, *It Makes You Sick – The Politics of the NHS*, Pluto Press, London, 1982.

Towler, Jean and Bramall, Joan, *Midwives in History and Society*, Croom Helm, Beckenham, UK, 1986.

Townsend, Peter and Davidson, Nick, *Inequalities in Health – The Black Report & The Health Divide*, Penguin Books, 1990.

Index

Health titles from Scarlet Press

They Said I Was Dead
The Complete Alternative Cure for Addiction

Anne McManus

Whatever your addiction – alcohol, cigarettes, pills or food – this book offers a new approach to recovery, one that is compelling, hard-hitting and effective. Drawing on her own experience of collapse, from PhD student of politics to addict of tranquillisers and alcohol, Anne McManus describes her decline and recovery through a mix of personal history and political analysis, set against the background of the shifts in left politics and thinking since 1968. Fierce and inspirational, her method includes understanding the reasons for low self-esteem, developing positive thinking, diet, exercise, yoga and meditation. And her book shows the pleasures a life free of addiction can give.

1 85727 091 6 pb / 1 85727 086 X hb

Lesbians Talk (Safer) Sex

Sue O'Sullivan and Pratibha Parmar

"A thoughtful and thorough contribution to the lesbians and HIV/AIDS debate." *Time Out*

"Excellent... this book is thoroughly essential reading." *Bad Attitude*

The need for safer sex has revolutionised sexual practice and its discussion within the gay male community and produced a series of hotly contested debates among lesbians which run far deeper than the issue of safer sex itself. Do lesbians need to think about safer sex at all? How are lesbians at risk from HIV? What has discussion of safer sex revealed about lesbian sexual practices in general? How have HIV and AIDS affected different lesbian communities? And how can lesbians develop a collective response to the AIDS crisis? Sue O'Sullivan and Pratibha Parmar discuss the issues with an international group of HIV and AIDS workers, sex educators and interested lesbians.

1 85727 020 7 pb

In the same series:

Lesbians Talk Queer Notions by Cherry Smyth

1 85727 025 8